To my sister Janet (1957–2024) who lived with Parkinson's disease.
I so wish you could have walked with me more.

Walk This Way

Practical walking ideas for fitness, health and happiness

Gill Stewart

BLOOMSBURY SPORT

LONDON · OXFORD · NEW YORK · NEW DELHI · SYDNEY

BLOOMSBURY SPORT
Bloomsbury Publishing Plc
50 Bedford Square, London, WC1B 3DP, UK
Bloomsbury Publishing Ireland Limited,
29 Earlsfort Terrace, Dublin 2, D02 AY28, Ireland

A catalogue record for this book is available from the British Library

Library of Congress Cataloguing-in-Publication data has been applied for

ISBN: TPB: 978-1-3994-1618-4; eBook: 978-1-3994-1617-7; ePDF: 978-1-3994-1619-1

2 4 6 8 10 9 7 5 3 1

Typeset in Minion by Deanta Global Publishing Services, Chennai, India
Printed and bound in Great Britain by Clays Ltd, Elcograf S.p.A.

To find out more about our authors and books visit www.bloomsbury.com and sign up for
our newsletters

For product safety related questions contact productsafety@bloomsbury.com

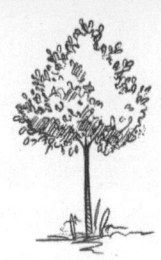

Contents

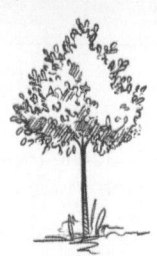

Introduction

Walking can be life-changing, and the purpose of *Walk This Way* is to reveal the power of a daily walk to improve your fitness, health and happiness. Whether you are new to walking or a seasoned hiker, my aim is to ensure that you gain something from every walk you take.

Our bodies may be designed to walk, but walking is far more than a method of getting from A to B. Each chapter of this book contains in-depth information about a different aspect of walking. I give you practical advice on how to enhance your natural posture and awareness to gain the most from every stride (see Chapter 1); what to wear and carry to stay safe and comfortable (see Chapter 8); and how to stay motivated (see Chapter 9).

I also guide you through the many mental health benefits of a daily walk; explore how you can connect with the great outdoors (see Chapter 3); and share a mix of mindfulness practices (see Chapter 2), fitness exercises (see Chapters 5 and 6) and daily inspirations (see Chapter 10).

Some of my suggestions are simple, others might need some forward-planning and a few are completely spontaneous, but all are worth trying! You'll find a range of quotes, testimonials and tips to inspire you along the way, and if you're after a more structured approach, then I have advice on creating a plan to support your walking as well (see the Appendix).

Why walk this way?

We all know that walking is good for us, but in case you need a reminder, the physical benefits of walking can include an improved immune system; better circulation, heart and lung function; joint flexibility and stronger muscles and bones. It can also promote weight loss; lower cholesterol; and reduce the risk of health conditions such as high blood pressure, diabetes, stroke, certain cancers, such as bladder, bowel and breast cancer, arthritis, and Alzheimer's disease.

That's on the physical side, but the mental health benefits can be just as compelling. Walking can aid sleep; increase energy; reduce stress and anxiety (walking for at least 2.5 hours a week reduces the risk of depression by up to 25 per cent); help memory and cognitive function; and boost mood and confidence levels. Given all that, it's hard to see why, if you're able to walk, you wouldn't!

About me

Before we begin, I thought I'd tell you a little about myself and my passion for walking. As a child I was very active and always wanted to be outdoors. As an adult I've done marathons, triathlons and endurance events, and have been involved in the fitness industry since the 1980s, which means I've seen pretty much every fitness fad there is going, sometimes two or three times!

During the years I spent running leisure centres and health clubs, I developed programmes that made exercise accessible and fun. I was one of the first women weight-training instructors in the UK and set up one of the earliest exercise referral programmes for those with medical conditions or poor health who needed to get active, and I also trained as a sports therapist and aromatherapist.

It was when I was living in Chamonix in the French Alps that I had a revelation about walking. I walked more because driving and parking were difficult, and the alpine location meant I had to do a lot of uphill walking. Despite not 'exercising' as I used to, I found I was fitter and healthier, even though I was organising my daily walk around work, chores and visitors. I also found I noticed my environment and the changing seasons more, and realised that balancing physical exertion with breathing, mindfulness and yoga in the wild flower meadows meant that I was working my body holistically.

Since 2008, I have created walking-based programmes for fitness and wellness, and run a national walking club called WALX. We call walking that improves your mind and body in a holistic way 'total body walking', and we encourage people to be active and motivate them to try new things.

My team and I have been teaching these programmes for several years, and we meet a lot of people who think walking is a waste of time, because they don't consider it to be exercise. They are usually there as part of a workplace group or for a 'discovery session' and we marvel at how these reluctant joiners subsequently think the programme is one of the most valuable activity sessions they have ever done.

That's how I want this book to make you feel, too, but please feel free to use it in whatever way you like. You can read each chapter in order or, once you've grasped the basics (see Chapter 1), you can dip in and out. However, you'll need to be ready to expand your horizons, so make sure you've got an open mind, a notebook and comfortable shoes.

I have put some resources on my website, including videos to demonstrate the standing yoga poses in Chapter 2, which you can access on the following link: walk-this-way-gill-stewart.walx.co.uk.

So, come and walk with me to discover for yourself how effective walking is as an exercise technique and how powerful it can be for both your physical and mental health. Without further ado, it's time to *Walk This Way*.

Accessibility and enjoying the great outdoors

While I build my exercises around walking on two feet, I would hate those who find that action difficult to miss out on the health and well-being benefits of this book, so if you currently get around with a frame, wheels or any other form of mobility support, please feel free to adapt the content to suit you.

'Walking is man's best medicine'
– Hippocrates

Glossary of the terms used in this book

Total body walking: A balanced, holistic way of using your daily steps to improve your body and mind. If you like following a specific routine, see the Appendix for how to build walking into your daily life and create your own total body walking plan.

Three elements of fitness: The three different ways you can (and should) work your body according to all health guidelines. They are cardiovascular (CV) fitness; strength and tone; and balance, flexibility and range of movement (see Chapter 4 for the theory behind each element, then follow the basic practical exercises for all-round fitness in Chapter 5 and advanced moves in Chapter 6).

Fitness walking sequences: Simple exercise sequences that incorporate all three elements of fitness (see above) that your body needs. Use the fitness walking sequences in Chapter 5 as a fun way to build strength, balance and a range of movement into your walking, to add variety, and challenge your mind and body.

Daily inspirations: Themed ideas that will add value to a walk, perfect for when you need a reason or some motivation to step outside. Pick and choose from the daily inspirations in Chapter 10 to suit your mood, needs or plans, or tailor them to the seasons, traditions or weather throughout the year.

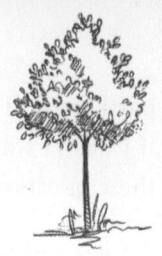

WALK THIS WAY...
For better posture and balance

Do you know how to walk? You've been doing it all your life, so of course you do, but do you know how to 'walk well'? With the right posture? So that you move naturally, don't lose your balance or fall over? Don't worry, I promise you're not going to fall over, but to walk well it's essential to 'get off on the right foot', which means making sure you have the correct posture.

A good posture is the basis of effective, comfortable movement. It maximises the use of your muscles and minimises the chance of injury. In this chapter I'm going to talk you through how to assess and reset your posture, and how to hold that posture as you move, so when you walk you involve your whole body, engage your core and take long, confident strides. Believe me, a good understanding of posture and an awareness of how you move while walking will set you up for success, wherever you want to take your walking.

Posture

Step 1: Assessing your posture

I often start a walking class by asking the group to walk round in a circle. This helps me look for any gait issues or injuries, but it also makes the participants think about *how* they are walking. I then ask them to walk as if I wasn't watching and that's what I need you to do now. Then answer these questions and be really honest with yourself:

- Do you 'economise' on posture when moving around indoors? Perhaps you don't stand up straight when you move from the kitchen counter to the sink or table, but remain slightly bent over.
- Do you walk with purpose and posture or do you lapse into what I call 'the teenage boy'? This is an economic gait where the upper body slouches and the legs move almost at a shuffle?

It's all too easy to take a shortcut and both these habits are common. Sometimes we aren't even conscious of them. For example, rather than standing up between picking plates up from the table, we may stay bent over as we know we will be placing them back down. Similarly, it is common to economise with your walking gait, especially when using smartphones on the go.

Never too late

It's never too late – or too early – to start walking with good posture. As babies, we typically learn to walk at between 10 and 18 months old. We generally have our legs wide and our hands out in front or up quite high as we 'toddle about', leaning from foot to foot. However, as our balance improves we bring our hands down to our sides and we begin to walk with our feet closer together, but bad habits tend to kick in when we're teenagers. It's fascinating, though, to observe how people morph back into the stable stance, hand positions and shuffle steps of babies as they age.

Step 2: Resetting your posture

Stand straight and work up your body, checking each part and resetting your posture. Do this every day until good posture becomes a habit. Use a mirror if that makes it easier.

FIND YOUR BASE POSITION

- Start by placing your feet side by side and close together.

- Turn your heels outwards, but keep your toes together.
- Then turn your toes outwards as well, in line with your heels, so there is a gap between your feet.
- Your feet should now be parallel and directly below your hips. This is your perfect base position,

SORT OUT YOUR STABILISING POSITION

- In your base position, gently rock backwards and forwards, shifting your weight between your toes and heels.
- Gently reduce the rocking until you achieve a nice, stable position where your weight is distributed evenly between your big toe and heel.
- You should be standing on the flat areas of the soles of your feet and you should feel 'grounded'.

CHECK YOUR KNEES

- Gently bend your knees. Feel how this activates the muscles in the front of your thighs.
- Then straighten your legs and check your thigh muscles again.
- Repeat this action, making sure that once you straighten up you keep your knees 'soft' and not locked.

DISCOVER YOUR OPTIMUM PELVIS POSITION

- If you're using a mirror, turn to the side, so it's easier to view your pelvis.
- Make sure your hips are in line with each other and your buttocks are relaxed.
- Place one hand behind your back and rest the back of your hand across the top of your buttocks. Place the other hand on your lower stomach/pelvic area, with your fingers pointing downwards.
- Gently rock your pelvis and press lightly with your hand on the front of the body. Reduce the tilting movements until your fingertips are facing straight down to the ground and the front of your pelvis is flat.
- Check the curve of your spine with the other hand. We all have different spinal curves, but this should feel comfortable and perhaps more accentuated than normal.

LOOSEN YOUR ARMS AND SHOULDERS

- To loosen your shoulders, stand in your new lower-body stance with your arms hanging down at your sides.
- First, roll your shoulders forwards, pulling them up towards your ears and then back. Allow them to relax and drop down.
- Check your little fingers are in line with the side seams of your trousers (or if you don't have seams, where they would be). This opens up your chest and brings your shoulders into a non-stress position. You may find this difficult, because when we are stressed and tight, often due to working on screens, we tend to draw the shoulders up (which I liken to wearing the shoulders as earrings).
- When your shoulders are low and relaxed, you will find it easier to mobilise your neck and therefore hold your head correctly, in line with your centre of gravity. Bring your shoulders up towards your ears again and gently try to move your head from side to side, feeling how restricted it is.
- Repeat this exercise. Once the shoulders are low and relaxed, gently ease your head from side to side again. It will feel looser.

BE AWARE OF YOUR HEAD

You particularly need to concentrate on head position, because using screens and smartphones daily causes us to tilt our head forward from its natural position. As the head weighs nearly as much as a bowling ball, this is not good for your posture or the health of your upper body.

- Your chin should be parallel to the ground, not jutting forward or tilting upwards.
- Your ears should be directly over your shoulders, and not in front of them.

PERFORM A FINAL BODY SCAN

- Stand and check from your feet up to make sure nothing has lapsed while you've been working on other areas.
- Take a moment to feel this aligned yet relaxed posture, which you will need to reset to in many of the exercises throughout this book.

Step 3: Move with good posture

Staying in the same posture-reset position from step 2, mobilise each area from the feet up to enhance your stride and natural gait.

START WITH YOUR LEGS

- March on the spot, noticing how, when you bend your knee at a right angle to lift your foot off the ground, your ankle is set at a similar angle and is placed back on the ground quite flatly. I call this 'square movement' (and we will come back to this concept later).
- Next, walk forward two or three paces, maintaining this high-knee, flat-foot action. You will feel some leg activation, but your strides will be short and square.
- Return to standing position. Now lift one leg and gently swing it forwards and backwards, keeping it straight. Notice how, in comparison to the movement above, this fully mobilises your hip joint. Also notice how it activates your core.
- With this leg action in mind, take a step forward with a straighter leg, placing your heel on the ground first and then rolling through your foot on to your toes. Step forward a few paces and repeat this action with both legs.

Note: This works the whole leg from top to bottom as well as the foot.

'Think of your feet massaging the earth with every step!' – Thich Nhat Hanh

The aim here – and it becomes even more important when we begin to look at pace and performance – is to avoid square movements, but the angles at your knee and foot joints are now more like triangles than squares, and this fluid movement increases your stride length, improves your posture and reduces 'bounce'. Now you have mastered these leg actions, you are ready to look at the rest of the body, moving upwards to explore each area.

MOVE ON TO THE CORE

- Practise striding forward with a straighter leg, heel strike and foot roll action, paying attention to your core.
- As you push off from your toes, actively engage the core muscles as you did in step 2.

BRING IN THE ARMS

Perfecting a good walking arm swing is also about the joint angles. The main movement needs to be at the shoulder joint, and the arm needs to be relaxed and straight, not bent so much at the elbow that it forms a right angle.

- Take a minute to swing a straight arm from your shoulder while standing still, checking in with your core and feeling the freedom of the movement.
- Next, bend your arm and try to swing it, noting how this shortens the movement and disengages the core.

Note: The latter movement forms a triangle, while the former movement is square and boxy.

Walking an object on a string

To teach yourself good arm protocol, try walking with a small object on a short string. I use dog balls when I teach this exercise, so if you have one look no further! Otherwise, think of a yo-yo or similar on a piece of string about 15 to 20 cm long.

- Swing your arms, first in a stationary position and then when walking.
- In both phases, the ball or object should swing calmly and in line with your arm when you are using a straight arm powered by the shoulders.
- Try bending the arm even slightly and the ball loses that smooth momentum and becomes jerky and uncomfortable – as will your stride.

NOW START WALKING

People often think the answer to building their fitness while walking is to *pump* their arms, when in fact it is the opposite. Try the following and feel the difference:

- First, try walking with long flowing strides and foot roll, then introduce the swing from the shoulders. It should feel purposeful but *natural*. This is walking with good posture.
- Now try walking with a shorter arm swing and bent arm, noting how this affects your legs and freedom of movement. Bending your arms means you revert to a pumping action with shorter strides and increased effort for less forward movement.

Step 4: Pulling it all together

- Run through your postural reset from step 2 before starting to walk slowly and carefully, concentrating on a longer stride and foot roll while engaging your core.
- Once you feel as if you're walking with a nice foot plant, swing your arms from the shoulders as in step 3.
- Take a moment to assess how it feels. If you have managed to master the basics, you should feel relaxed but with good posture, your core engaged and long, confident strides. Your whole body should be involved in the action. If you don't feel this yet, don't worry, just keep running through each step until you do. It may take a while to feel totally natural, but keep practising.

Set a marker

Pick a short distance, perhaps between two trees or the length of a football pitch, and see how it becomes easier each day to maintain good walking form. It can help to count your strides, too, as you may find it takes you fewer steps to cover the distance as you get fitter and more proficient.

Bringing awareness to your natural movements

Another factor in maintaining good posture when you walk is understanding how our brains and body are interlinked when it comes to moving. Let's look at how we were designed to move. As hunter-gatherers, we probably walked between three and 10 miles a day. Much of this walking would have been up hills and down dales, and we would have needed to stay alert, on the look-out for food and predators. Nowadays, we have minimised our movements. Thanks to tarmacked footpaths we are more likely to walk on flat, even surfaces, and we frequently crane our necks, staring down at our smartphones, oblivious to the world around us. For longer distances we drive or use public transport, and it is rare for most people to cover 10 miles on foot in a day.

Although it's fine to walk on an even path, a treadmill or a running track, I think walking 'wildly' outdoors is the best way to boost total well-being as it's more natural for us. I have seen great improvements in the movement patterns and balance of regular walkers who have shifted from paved paths to something less predictable.

Because you need to focus more on your steps, walking outdoors on challenging terrain requires more physical effort, engages the core, improves joint flexibility and takes your mind away from the mundane. On uneven ground, before you place your feet and as you move, your mind and body must work very closely together to process a range of sensory information. This is called proprioception and it helps you respond to your environment. For example, if the surface you're walking on is more slippery than you thought, you might need to make a quick readjustment. You sense your position in relation to your surroundings and shift your centre of gravity, but you do it without conscious thought

Modern lifestyles mean we probably don't utilise these links between mind and body enough. Also, as we age, these links begin to diminish – especially if they are not used much – so a walk on the wild side is a great way to keep challenging them, helping you to stay on your feet into older age and avoid falls (see also the section on balance in Chapter 4, page 63).

Walking with your eyes closed

The visual information provided by your eyes is also crucial for walking. Pick a safe surface and have somebody on hand to guide you, then try walking with your eyes closed. You will soon realise how powerful the links are between your eyes, your brain and your muscles.

I've mentioned your centre of gravity a couple of times already, because it's essential to good posture and gait. The following exercises are designed to make you aware of how you were designed to move by utilising your centre of gravity. They can help you understand your posture and gait, and practise how to adjust them.

Centre of gravity exercises

Imagine walking over some stepping stones. You will immediately notice that you plant your feet with more care and adjust your body position each time you take a step. Your hands are likely to be out at the sides, too. The links between your brain and body automatically kick in to ensure you are balanced and less likely to fall. Exploring how arm position changes your centre of gravity is a great way to begin.

TRAY CARRY - ARMS TUCKED IN

- Stand with your feet together and arms bent at 90 degrees, elbows tucked in to your sides. Turn your palms to the floor – this stops you gripping – and imagine you are carrying a tray, with your arms in quite close to your body.
- Start walking and keep looking ahead, concentrating on your posture with your arms in this position.
- Take it further by trying to climb some steps or going up and down a hill.

'100 steps backwards are worth 1000 steps forwards' - Chinese proverb

Place something light, such as beanbags, on to the back of your hands. Try to walk smoothly enough so the beanbags don't slip off (it's harder than it sounds).

TRAY CARRY - ARMS STRAIGHT IN FRONT

- Repeat the exercise with your arms stretched out in front of you. Notice how you need to adjust your posture – pay attention to the natural curve of your spine. You may be tempted to lean forwards slightly, but don't.
- Try to keep your gait smooth and observe how your arm position can affect this.

TRAY CARRY - ARMS OUTSTRETCHED TO THE SIDES

- This exercise can also work with or without the beanbags/light objects mentioned above.
- Walk forwards, concentrating on your posture, then stretch your arms out to the sides.
- At first, you may want to lean backwards slightly or look down, which causes a slight forward lean. Notice how you adjust and walk taller once you become more aware of your posture.

TRAY CARRY - ARMS BEHIND YOU

- Repeat the process, now with your arms stretched out behind you.
- This stance should bring the most significant change to your initial posture. Watch out for the tendency to push your bottom out or stick your chest forward.
- Ensure you have a natural curve to your spine.

TRAY CARRY - ARMS ABOVE THE HEAD

- Repeat the process, this time with your arms raised above your head, close to your ears.
- At first you will tend to lean backwards (stiffness around the shoulders can cause this).

- Resist the temptation to look down instead of forwards, and notice how a change in head position can affect your posture. Use the posture reset (see page 12) to check your spine is in line.

Heavy headed

Your head is heavy. It weighs about 5kg (12lb) when you are holding it well, but if you increase the angle of tilt, you increase the 'weight' of your head and the work the rest of your body needs to do. Studies have shown that a tilt of about 15 degrees can increase the weight of your head to just under 14kg (30lb). Increase the tilt angle further to a 60-degree hunched position and the weight increases to about 27kg (60lb). Text neck is a major issue among those who use devices constantly and it puts pressure on the spine.

Change of direction exercises

The following exercises build on the waiter or tray carry, but bring in changes of direction and turns – all things you will encounter on wilder walks and that we are designed to do, but often don't. The aim is to think about posture as you perform each of these exercises.

DIRECTIONAL CHANGES AROUND A POST OR TREE

- Mark out a short route with a post or small tree at each end – poles are great for this, too.
- Walk from one to the other, walk around the far post or tree and return, keeping a good posture.
- After you have walked in both directions, attempt to walk around the post or tree with your back towards it, before switching to face the other post or tree and walking towards it.
- Repeat at both ends a couple of times.
- Finally, repeat the exercise above, but (ensuring you are safe) walk backwards for a few steps towards the other post or tree before turning fully to face it.

DIRECTIONAL CHANGES AROUND OBJECTS ON THE GROUND

- Place a marker on the ground and walk 40 paces before placing another marker in line with the first.
- Walk from one marker to the other, crossing over at the midpoint so you are walking in a figure of eight, circling round the markers at each end. It sounds easy, but keeping good walking form and posture while you switch direction is key.

Backwards walking

Backwards walking is incredibly powerful, because it brings together the two aspects of walking that we've been discussing in this chapter – good posture and improving our awareness of the way we move. In Japan, walking backwards is a popular way to exercise outdoors, with claims that it can burn 10 times more calories than forwards walking. The larger muscles that are engaged and the unusual movement pattern add to the exercise effect, and it certainly increases the cardiovascular effects of every step (as outlined in a study where it was used to measure changes in body composition), but I would not advocate it as the new super-diet. I do, however, think it's something we should all do as part of a holistic way of working the body, improving balance and stimulating the brain, which has to work harder to cope with the fact you can't see where you are going.

What are the benefits of backwards walking?

- It engages the backside, front of the thighs, shins, ankles and lesser-used muscles in the feet.
- It reduces the forces that go through the knees and lower back, and can alleviate back pain when practised regularly.
- It encourages you to stand taller and improve your posture.
- It improves flexibility, especially if you are sedentary.
- It helps with coordination and balance.

- It can help with recall, as it's thought walking backwards may also help your mind retrace its thoughts.
- It helps reduce stress on the joints.
- It boosts brain health, improving response time and decision-making.
- It improves gait when practised regularly.
- It uses more energy than forwards walking.

Why is backwards walking so effective?

Because you have to reach backwards and plant with the toes or ball of the foot to perform your foot roll, you are working the *front* of the legs rather than the calves (which are used more often), thus reducing the impact of the foot strike on the knees. This backwards action also engages the buttock and quadriceps muscles more, which encourages you to stand taller. This, coupled with a backward swing of the leg, helps to lengthen the hip flexor muscles, which do tend to get tight if you sit down for long periods, often causing back pain.

Backwards walking is a remarkable recovery and fitness building tool. As a sports therapist, I often used it for those recovering from lower-body injuries in their knees, hips, back, groin or Achilles tendon. Coaches include backwards jogging in training for sports where frequent changes of direction might occur, not simply because the sportsman may need to move backwards, but because of the way it works the joints and any underused muscles. It's also a great exercise inclusion for active ageing – simple to do (as long as safety has been considered) and accessible to most people. In fact, US professors Janet Dufek and Barry Bates studied the benefits on back and lower joint pain for 40 years and reinforced its value for older adults and falls prevention.

How do I try it?

Backwards walking can be performed indoors and outdoors. Get used to adding phases of backwards walking into your routine whenever appropriate. See the backwards walking sequence (page 98) for further practice.

START INDOORS

- Practise planting the foot and stepping back indoors alongside a rail or row of cabinets.
- Use a treadmill with a side handrail (I do not advise backwards walking on a treadmill with no supporting rails).

VENTURE OUTDOORS

- Make sure you have a clear path or have somebody spot for you.
- Hold both hands with a partner when facing each other and take turns to walk forwards or backwards in a push-me-pull-you action.
- Start *slowly* and walk for a minute or two at first. Add a minute each time you practise, if you can.

TIP

Look for rails to hold on to while you are backwards walking out and about – in some parks these are being installed to help people with balance or walking difficulties.

Now you have mastered how to walk with good posture and awareness, in the next chapter we'll explore how to use walking to improve your mental health and well-being.

2

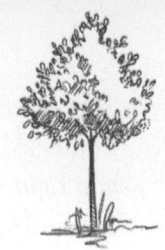

WALK THIS WAY...
To better mental health

The simple act of walking is a powerful mood-booster, and being outdoors, breathing fresh air and moving are great ways to improve your mental health. Exercise is known to raise levels of the feel-good hormone, serotonin, and reduce levels of the stress hormone, cortisol, but if you want to get active you don't have to go striding out at top speed. There are real benefits to slowing down, and walking at a much slower pace will stimulate your brain function and sharpen your focus.

While you're out walking, I'll show you how to add to those benefits with some mindfulness practices to empty your mind, and some breathing exercises, to encourage your body to relax. In this chapter I also suggest you incorporate some standing yoga postures into your daily walk, so I'm passing on the ones that work for me. They will not only improve your flexibility, strength and stability, but also increase your awareness of your body, which will make you more conscious of how you move.

Mindfulness practices

Be present

Let's start with a simple way to clear the mind. The first thing you should do when using walking to help you de-stress is to be *present in the moment*.

- Take a deep breath, step out and encourage yourself to be immersed in your surroundings and what is happening around you *right now*.
- Remind yourself to not think of the past, the awful day you may have had or what you need to do later.
- Learn to use your senses. Note the weather conditions and how they make you feel. Is the wind buffeting you? Is there sun on your back? Are you warm or cold?
- Who and what else is out with you today? Look for people, dogs, birdsong and traffic. Imagine what they are doing to take the focus away from your thoughts.
- If your mind comes back to unpleasant thoughts, worry or the past and future, train yourself to be in the moment again.

Focus on your body

Directing your attention to your body and how it's moving will help to declutter the mind.

- Reset your posture (see page 12) and start walking. Concentrate on how your body *feels* as you walk.
- Breathe deeply as you take each step – matching breaths to steps can help (see 4 x 4 breathing on page 27).
- Think about the heel-to-toe action of your feet as they 'massage the ground.' Focus on the muscles and bones in your feet, keeping you upright and stable.
- Concentrate on your legs, feeling the muscles tense and relax as they move through each step.
- Think about your hips as each leg moves back and forth, and the core as it engages as you push off with your toes.
- Consider whether your steps are slow and heavy or light and free. Explore both.
- Study the terrain you are covering and think about how it feels and sounds beneath your feet. Come up with words to describe it – soft, slippery, squelchy, dusty.
- If you notice that your attention has drifted or you are becoming caught up in everyday thoughts, gently bring your mind back by

focusing again on your feet and the simple action of them hitting the ground.

Concentrate on your breathing

A great way to clear your mind is to learn breathwork. The following two practices help with this.

4 X 4 BREATHING

This a great walking-based breathing exercise.

- Practise breathing in time with your steps.
- Inhale deeply through your nose for a count of four, trying to expand your stomach as well as your chest. Imagine you have a balloon in your lower abdomen and try to allow the breath to flow deeper than usual to inflate that balloon.
- Hold that breath in for a count of four (if you can).
- Expel the air fully through your mouth for a count of four.
- Once you have exhaled, wait a count of four before breathing in again and repeating.

Now try matching your breathing to your walking pace.

- Walk at a steady pace and wait until you have got into your stride, then inhale deeply for two paces.
- Hold that breath in for two paces.
- Exhale for two paces.
- Relax as you breathe and keep doing this for as long as you feel comfortable.

TIP

It's a good idea to practise deeper breathing in daily life rather than just doing it as a walking exercise.

Chandrika did not leave her house for three years, but then plucked up the courage to join a walking group.

'I have never met such lovely people and I have never been outside in nature so much. I have gone from an unfit asthmatic who struggled to walk a mile to somebody who is not breathless and is even tackling hills with the support of the group. I actually think it's all down to confidence and that I used the breathing as an excuse before. This has literally changed my life! Walking is like a drug! I'm actually addicted to it and it makes me happier than I have been for a long time. My friends and family have noticed the difference, too.'

3-4-5 BREATHING

This exercise can be practised daily at home, as well as on a walk. It is an age-old yoga technique that works on the basis that if your exhale is longer than your inhale, it reduces your stress state and encourages your body to relax.

- Stop in a suitable place, and before you start make sure you are breathing normally and are not 'puffed out' after walking briskly or climbing a hill.
- Inhale for a count of three.
- Hold that breath in for a count of four.
- Exhale for a count of five.
- Repeat this a couple of times and when you feel comfortable doing it, work towards extending each phase.

'Solvitur ambulando – it is solved by walking'

Slow down to encourage brain function

Walking at a slower pace has been proven to connect your mind and body; to encourage your brain function, concentration and focus.

(Walking at a brisker pace, on the other hand, clears your mind to focus on walking itself and improving your body's performance.)

As a fitness professional and former runner, I never used to understand the 'amblers' I met on the footpaths. I thought they would benefit more if they upped their pace – surely, they would need to be out all day to cover any distance at all! – and I didn't appreciate what they were gaining.

Now, however, I realise that we were designed to walk almost continually most days, but at a varied pace. Hunter-gatherers may have needed to move quickly to locate prey or food, but they had to slow down to identify, stalk and catch that prey.

Experience the benefits of slow walking for yourself by going for a walk, starting off at your usual pace and then, midway through, consciously dropping your pace. At first, you may feel frustrated – potentially even awkward – but after a while you will fall into a rhythm and that's when your mind will begin to wander.

Writers and artists describe how when they slow down their creativity kicks in, so be patient and alert to how different you might feel when walking slowly. Many of my daily inspirations (see Chapter 10) involve periods of slowness, because I believe it is one of the most fundamental ways to use walking to improve mental health.

The science backs this up

In Praise of Walking is one of the best books on walking I've ever read. In it, the neuroscientist Shane O'Mara explains just how walking is linked to brain function, memory, learning and even natural navigation. His explanation of theta brainwaves will encourage you to find your natural walking rhythm. Theta is a pulse or frequency (7–8Hz, to be precise) that happens when walking, which has a powerful effect on brain function. Similarly, he describes how brain-derived neurotrophic factor, a kind of molecular fertiliser produced in the brain when we're walking, can help improve our response to the process of ageing and address the damage caused by trauma or infection.

Standing yoga poses to use while out walking

Yoga – the ultimate mind and body exercise – works wonderfully when combined with a walk, where you can add fresh air, gentle cardio-vascular exercise and the power of nature to the mix. However, it's probably best to stick to standing poses to avoid getting muddy or having to carry a mat.

I am not a yoga teacher, but I have had many positive experiences with yoga over the years, and I add selected relaxing and lengthening poses into my total body walking plan. My favourites are those that encourage relaxation, improve flexibility and stimulate major organs.

Here I have deliberately selected some simple, empowering poses. Each has its own benefits and mastering just a few can help boost your immune system and general health, so pick and choose or combine them into a simple flowing sequence.

Yoga works best when you are breathing evenly, feel calm and are nicely warmed up. I recommend incorporating the poses after you have walked for at least 10 minutes. Step off the path into a quiet spot, because a calm place will add to the calming effect. Hold the poses for between 30 and 60 seconds or up to five breaths, depending on how you feel, your balance, the time available and how warm it is.

If it's a cool day, pick shorter poses and perform them with more speed, but take the time to luxuriate in long, slow poses if it's balmy outside. If the weather is extremely cold, leave the poses until the end of the walk and include them in your cool-down, as it's not advisable to get cold mid-walk.

I am delighted to share my favourite poses with you and I hope they will inspire you to explore this ancient practice more deeply.

'Yoga is a combination of physiotherapy, psychotherapy and spiritual therapy' – B.K.S. Iyengar

While it's great to take your shoes and socks off so you can engage with the earth, don't let keeping them on stop you practising these poses. It's not always practical to discard the shoes mid-walk, but it's always worth stopping for a quick pose.

Safety first

Always work at your own level. If something feels uncomfortable or unnatural, stop and check that you are performing the pose correctly. If you have any back, joint or balance conditions, do not attempt these poses outdoors without prior guidance from a professional and plenty of practice.

Mountain pose (*Tadāsana*)

Everything starts with the Mountain pose – a great way to ground yourself and connect with nature before moving on to other poses.

- Stand with your feet shoulder-width apart. Wiggle your toes and – if your shoes allow – lift and spread your toes before ensuring your whole foot is placed naturally on the ground.
- Push into your feet as you gently allow the crown of your head to rise, stretching out your spine and pulling up through the front of your legs with your chin parallel to the floor.
- Do not tighten or lift your shoulders – they should be relaxed.
- Let your arms hang by your sides with your palms facing forwards.
- Take time to notice your breathing, which should be natural. Take a deep breath, and imagine the fresh air filling your lungs and energising your body. Exhale slowly through your mouth as you enjoy the feeling of the earth beneath your feet.

To add value to a Mountain pose, take a look at the breathing exercises (pages 27 and 28) and the invitation to greet the sun or moon (page 43).

Tree pose (*Vrikshāsana*)

This pose activates the muscles in your legs, ankles and feet, and improves balance, which will help when walking on uneven terrain. It flows naturally on from Mountain pose and I love that they both connect you to the world around you.

- Start in Mountain pose (see page 31), lifting yourself up so you feel nice and tall.
- Rotate one knee out to the side, lifting your heel off the floor.
- Check in with your balance. If you are comfortable, place the sole of your lifted foot against the ankle of your anchor leg, keeping your knee turned out.
- Move your lifted foot to just below your knee and hold this position.
- Keep your hands in front of you in a prayer position, out to the sides or raised above your head. Do what feels comfortable for you and, as you improve, explore different arm positions.
- Repeat the posture, lifting the other leg instead.

Half lift (*Ardha Uttanāsana*)

This pose releases the hamstrings, lengthens the calf muscles and opens the chest to allow for deeper breathing – all beneficial when out on a walk.

- Start in Mountain pose (see page 31).
- Gently roll down through your spine with your hands on your thighs until you are bent forward at the waist.
- Keep your weight on the balls of your feet and your knees bent.
- Gently extend your arms forward while trying to maintain a flat back.

- If you can, lengthen through your legs, again trying to maintain lengthening through your spine and reaching your arms out.
- Keeping your weight forward, gently come out of the lift, softening your knees to roll up through your spine and come back to Mountain pose.

TIP

Keeping your arms close to your ears will make the half lift slightly more difficult.

Forward fold pose (*Uttanāsana*)

This pose increases your range of motion in the spine, hips, knees and ankles. By encouraging you to put more weight on the balls of your feet, it also improves posture.

- Start in Mountain pose (see page 31) with your feet rooted to the ground.
- Reach up to the sky, stretching your body right up into your fingertips.
- Take a breath in and, when you are ready to exhale, drop into a loose and free-flowing forward fold.
- Your neck should be relaxed and your arms hanging loosely to the sides.
- You may want to bend your knees slightly or move each leg into a straighter position – whatever feels comfortable for your back.
- Gently curl back up to Mountain pose, with your feet pushing into the ground as you breathe naturally.

TIP

If you are stiff through your back you may want to start by practising the half lift before folding all the way.

Twisting chair pose (*Parivrtta Utkatāsana*)

This pose strengthens the core, back, hips, legs, glutes and ankles. It also helps to improve balance and coordination, aiding focus and stability.

- Start in Mountain pose (see page 31), exhale and gently squat down to a comfortable 'sitting position' (imagine there is a chair beneath you).
- Keep your hands either close to your body or extended out in front of you.
- Lengthen through your spine. Keep your knees together and chest open.
- Gently rotate, so the back of one hand is on the outside of the opposite knee with the other hand raised above you.
- Look up towards the top hand (if you can), before coming back to the centre and rolling back up through your spine to Mountain pose.
- Repeat on the opposite side.

Warrior poses

Warrior poses are beneficial for strength, stability and balance. Once you have mastered Warrior 1, you can try the two variations: Warrior 2 and Reverse warrior.

WARRIOR 1 (*VIRABHADRĀSANA I*)

Warrior 1 strengthens the lower body and increases flexibility in the hips.

- From Mountain pose (see page 31), step back with your right foot and rotate that foot out to the right side, ensuring you are comfortable through the hip.
- Your left toes should remain facing the front, with knees bent but still in line with the hip (not extending out past the toes).
- Reach your hands forward with your palms facing each other.
- If you can, raise your arms above your head, opening your chest and looking up to the sky.
- Gently bring your arms back down to your sides and step your right foot back into position for Mountain pose.
- Repeat with the left leg.

WARRIOR 2 (*VIRABHADRĀSANA II*)

Warrior 2 increases blood flow to the legs and groin, and strengthens the leg muscles.

- Take a step to one side with your feet at right angles to each other.
- Extend your arms to the sides and hold them outstretched, ideally at shoulder height.
- Return your arms to the centre and then return to Mountain pose (see page 31).
- Repeat on the opposite side.

REVERSE WARRIOR (*VIPARITA VIRABHADRĀSANA*)

This pose stretches the groin, hips, legs and obliques.

- Repeat Warrior 2, but continue with a final stretch. Take your forward arm, with your palm facing upwards, up to the sky (keep your arm close to your cheek).
- Lower your outstretched rear arm so your hand can rest on your rear leg.
- Gently return to Warrior 2, then lower your arms and return to Mountain pose (see page 31).
- Repeat on the opposite side.

Triangle pose (*Trikonāsana*)

This pose boosts balance and stability, and improves flexibility by strengthening the chest, arms, legs and ankles. It can also improve focus by reducing stress.

- Start with Warrior 2, raising your arms to shoulder height as before.
- Next, push the ground away with your feet as you gently lower your front arm to rest on your bent leg.
- Raise your back arm up to the sky.
- Keep everything in line by imagining you are between two panes of glass. Straighten your front leg, then your arm, so your hand lowers towards your calves or ankles.

- You may find you want to look up to the sky or down at the floor – you can choose, as long as you form a beautiful triangle.
- Repeat on the opposite side.
- Return to Mountain pose.

To check out a short video of each of these poses, scan this QR code or visit walk-this-way-gill-stewart.walx.co.uk:

> **TIP**
>
> If you enjoy the mobility and well-being you get from these poses and are ready to get on the ground in a kneeling position, look up the Cat and Cow poses, which are fantastic for your lower back.

If you're new to yoga you may find it helpful to attend a class to refine the poses and, in particular, the breathing, but whatever your previous experience, do please do take the time to explore these mindfulness practices and yoga poses. Along with a deeper connection with nature, which is what we're going to explore next, I am confident that they will enhance your walking and give you the skills to manage mood, anxiety and stress.

'The best remedy for a short temper is a long walk' – Jacqueline Schiff

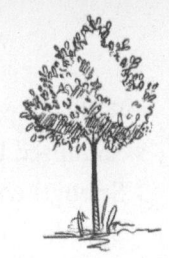

CHAPTER

3

WALK THIS WAY...
To connect with nature

It's often used to encourage people to get outside more, but what does the phrase 'connecting with nature' actually mean? Those who practise the Japanese art of *Shinrin-yoku* (forest bathing) use the term 'immersion in nature'. This is a slightly different and useful way of framing it, because rather than simply walking past or through nature, we need to practise how we can become at one with it; how we can bathe or immerse ourselves in it.

This chapter looks at the many benefits of getting outside more and why connecting with nature has such a positive effect on us. It then explains how to reconnect with nature by engaging all your senses and outlines a series of practices that will enable you to deepen your connection.

The benefits of connecting with nature

By connecting deeply with nature, we can enjoy:

- Reduced anxiety
- Improved mood
- Increased energy
- Better sleep
- Improved cognitive performance

- Reduced pain
- Stabilised blood pressure
- Strengthened immune system
- Speedier recovery from injury and illness

Why does connecting with nature have such a positive effect?

Connecting with nature feels right and it feels relaxing. That's because it's in our DNA and is as necessary for our survival as breathing. We may have evolved to live in urban environments and use vehicles, but we still have that deep need to stay connected to other species, to the seasons and to the natural world in general. This is often referred to as 'biophilia', a term first coined in 1984 by an American biologist called Edward O. Wilson, and since then there have been numerous studies looking at biophilia in relation to building design, rewilding, healing, mental health and many other areas of human existence.

'When you have heard the meadowlark and caught the scent of fresh-ploughed earth, peace cannot escape you' – Sequichie Comingdeer

NATURAL CHEMICALS FROM TREES HAVE A POSITIVE IMPACT AT A CELLULAR LEVEL

Japanese scientists recently discovered that people who walked in a cedar forest as opposed to a city or laboratory had lower levels of cortisol, and that the aromatic essential oils emitted by the trees (called phytoncides) also caused biological changes in the body. As an aromatherapist, this does not surprise me. And when later studies revealed that the essential oils from cedars boost our natural killer cells, even when they're pumped into a hotel room, it reinforced why a walk in the forest is so beneficial. Plants produce these chemicals to ward off insects, so it makes sense that we can use them to fight off tumours and infections.

WE FEEL AT EASE WITH NATURAL SHAPES

We are made up of cells, just like all other living organisms. A good way to remind ourselves of this is to conjure up the shape of a tree, where a central stem leads to branches and then smaller twigs. This pattern appears consistently in nature, including inside our lungs. From the veins on the backs of leaves to a cauliflower cross-section, from hexagonal honeycomb to spirals in a cut tree trunk, and from conical pine cones to the underground mycelium network that connects plants and trees, there are so many patterns in nature. Unlike the regular, hard-edged urban landscapes many of us live and work in, they make sense to our brains. That's why we love to look at art that uses these natural shapes, whether it's flowers, shells, landscapes or the human form.

Of course, nature is beautiful too, so looking at it directly affects our emotions, making us feel relaxed and evoking a smile. I like to watch how people behave when they reach a viewpoint, because what starts with a 'wow' tends to change to a silence and then a deep sigh as they are affected by what they are looking at.

NATURE GIVES US A SENSE OF AWE

Nature makes us feel less significant. Imagine looking at the Grand Canyon, a view from a mountaintop or the wild power of a waterfall. The feeling of awe you will experience is so grounding. I think that's why walking in wilder places like mountains can be so life-changing and addictive. I also think you can find awe in something as simple as a flower, if you take the time to look at it closely enough.

Gaining a connection with nature is proven to increase our desire to protect the world for future generations. It changes our approach to many areas of our lives, from what we eat and the way we dispose of things to how we travel. This often has a direct effect on both our mental and physical health. Once you begin to experience how climate change is affecting the rivers, plants, flowers, birdsong and insects on your walks, it makes it more real.

RECONNECTING TO THE SEASONS HELPS US TO FEEL PART OF NATURE

Our busy lifestyles and reliance on technology have removed us from nature, traditional practices and a knowledge of what may feed or heal us, and what we should avoid. I'm not saying we should revert to a time when our nutrition, comfort and happiness all came from nature, but I do think we can tap into some of that knowledge and simple rhythm of life on our daily walks. You will notice how I draw on ancient cultures and wisdom for the daily inspirations (see Chapter 10).

'Everything's a circle. We're each responsible for our own actions. It will come back' – Betty Laverdure

How to reconnect with nature

I've mentioned how smelling natural essential oils and looking at natural shapes are beneficial, but it is important to think about your other senses as well if you want to learn how to maximise your immersion in nature as you walk. We may have forgotten how to do it, but connecting with nature is about using our senses in the way they were designed to be used. You may need to learn to stop – even sit – for a while to get the full benefits, but the skills you will learn will be transferable to any walk you do in the future.

The Japanese art of *Shinrin-yoku*

On a *Shinrin-yoku* (forest bathing) session, the aim is to take the time to fully immerse yourself in nature. It's about slowing down, and ensuring you relax and stay long enough to let go of day-to-day thoughts, while breathing in the healing forest air. You might be invited to listen intensely to the sounds around you and look more deeply into what is moving, the colours and the light. Concentrating on them and using the senses of smell and touch to explore things in more detail enhances the connection with nature, taking us back to our natural state and removing us from the day to day.

Invitation practice 1: Engage the senses

Sight gives our brains so much information that we tend to rely on it. This invitation helps you to heighten the other senses instead.

During your walk, find a safe place away from outside noise and surrounded by nature – ideally trees. If you are alone, it's best to choose a seat on a log or the ground (see soft seat pad on page 133). If you are with others, take turns to guide each other while standing or walking. Close your eyes and focus on each sense in turn (taste is explored later in the chapter – see page 46).

HEARING

This is a wonderful way to improve your awareness of the nature around you. Notice how sounds appear clearer when you can't see what surrounds you.

- Listen intently to the wind through the leaves, the dripping of the rain, birdsong, insects buzzing.
- Ask yourself what is happening around you. Was the twig cracking something passing by? Which way did that bird fly over? What is moving in the wind? How far away is the water trickling or dripping?
- Finally, note things that you might have missed had you been seeing everything as usual.

TOUCH

This is a great invitation to do with others, as sharing your chosen words afterwards can be very special.

- Keeping your eyes closed, use your hands to explore the forest floor around you and, if sitting, the log or stump.
- Feel the different textures and find a word that aptly describes them. Try not to focus on simple words like hard, soft, wet or cold.
- Think of how you might describe the texture to somebody else, using words such as rough, silky, spongy, sticky, shiny, crinkly, velvety and prickly.
- Notice how your mind clears of everything else as your brain processes what you are feeling and finds the appropriate word.

SMELL

Stop processing what you see and your sense of smell will become more acute. Once you have mastered taking in scents when sitting, you can continue to do so as you walk.

- Try to identify not only the smells of nature, but also specific scents, if you can.
- Name or describe them to yourself, using words such as musty, sharp, tangy, fragrant or sweet.

Invitation practice 2: Breathe with a tree

This invitation is profound; while breath work and breathing exercises are powerful, for me this is the ultimate way to feel part of nature. It will involve a stop en route, but I guarantee you will want to practise it more than once. It is a powerful way to realise how we need the sun and nature to survive, and you will feel a deep connection with the tree.

- Sit quietly with your back touching the trunk of a favourite tree, or a tree you feel connected to, and close your eyes. As you breathe in and out, be aware of the trunk against your body.
- Look down at its roots and, as you breathe in slowly, let your eyes move upwards into the canopy. Inhale deeply, thinking about the good clean oxygen you are taking deep into your lungs each time you breathe in.
- Hold the breath briefly and think about how your body will use the oxygen for energy and life.
- Breathe out slowly, thinking about how you are expelling the by-products of that activity within your body. The creation of energy within our cells produces carbon dioxide and we breathe out much more than we inhale.
- Continue for a few breath cycles, focusing on the tree as you do so.
- Every time you breathe in the clean oxygen, thank the tree for helping it be that way – imagine how the tree also 'breathes' this out as it uses the sun and carbon dioxide to create its own energy via photosynthesis. Think of it flowing through the air from the tree to you and how it is nurturing you.

- As you exhale, imagine the carbon dioxide flowing out of your lungs and the tree thanking you for it. Picture it being taken in via the leaves to produce the strong, sturdy and wonderful specimen that you are leaning against.
- Take a moment to reflect how important all living things are as part of our world.
- Continue to breathe with the tree. You will feel a connection and calmness that is so powerful and special.

Once you have mastered this practice sitting, you can employ this exercise as you walk, too.

Invitation practice 3: Greet the sun or moon

Although most of us can gasp 'wow' when we see a nice view, it is possible to work on this emotive response to nature. Many of the daily inspirations – from listening to a dawn chorus to having fun with cloud and tree shapes – will do just that (see Chapter 10). However, there is one magical way to practise this and it's a simple but profound ritual found in yoga practice and performed by monks: greeting the sun or moon. If you practise this regularly, you will experience this transition more profoundly.

- Look up the time the sun will rise tomorrow morning and set your alarm to go off before it does.
- Venture outside, or ideally head off for a walk in the darkness, and position yourself so you will see the sun appear on the horizon. (You will need a fairly clear day.)
- Watch the sun emerge as a tiny slither and grow into a semi-circle, noticing the light changing and the affect it has on the world around you.
- Greet it silently and thank it for making the flowers and crops grow, and for providing warmth and light. Take a moment to think about other creatures around you and how they are reacting to this transition from night to day. The essential oils in flowers are at their strongest as the day begins, snakes emerge to warm up and, of course, the birds sing.

- Wait until the sun is fully visible and the world is waking up around you and explore how emotionally connected you feel by taking this time to watch something that our forebears relied on and marvelled at, too. Remind yourself that others around the world will also see this daily and that no matter what problems or hardships any of us are facing, the sun can be relied on to be back again tomorrow.
- There are ways to maximise the effect, from standing barefoot on wet grass to using all your senses to observe the sunrise.

Replicate this process at the end of a day by connecting with the moon as it takes over. Supermoons can be magnificent, and it's grounding to imagine the force of the moon on our tides and the seasons. In the daily inspirations (see Chapter 10), I explain how our ancestors viewed each moon and it's great to understand how we worked in harmony with them. Watching the emergence of both the sun and the moon are humbling, emotional and unforgettable experiences.

Invitation practice 4: Hedgerow immersion

Here we not only employ the basic senses, but also learn how to see things around us differently and gain a deeper understanding of nature. I invite you to get to know your local hedges and to take time to look at what's growing and living inside them. Remind yourself not to simply walk past them, but to settle in beside them and be constantly aware of the changes happening every day. You will be glad you did.

Hedges are a living ecosystem, full of life, nutritional benefit, scent, beauty, seasonal changes and even historical interest. They weave a story about our ancestors, shape the landscape around us and are a great way to learn how to apply this 'deep dive' into nature and a sensory approach to everything you see when out walking. Give it a go – it's for any walker, urban or rural.

- Walk along a track bordered by hedges with a stunning view ahead. Your eyes will be drawn to the view, and you may even stop and smell the air or feel the sun on your back. All of these are valuable practices and will make you feel good, but I urge you to slow down and think about using *all* your senses.

- It is easy to consider the hedgerow as you might a fence or wall – simply a boundary that keeps you on track – unless you take the time to use all your senses and consider it as a living ecosystem.
- Take time to *touch* the leaves and *smell* the flowers. *Listen* to the birds and *watch* the tiny insects.
- Step back and consider the age and position of the hedge – is it fairly new and part of a modern development or an ancient boundary steeped in history? Many hedgerows have helped to shape the landscape, which makes them a great navigational tool.
- One of my favourite things to do is to learn how to identify everyday plants and understand how many can provide us with nutrition and delicious drinks. Here, your sense of taste can add another dimension once you know what is safe to enjoy.

Poems and paintings

- -

I love old poems and paintings that describe and depict the wonder of landscapes, particularly hedgerows, reinforcing the importance of sharing our space with nature. Cicely Mary Barker accurately describes the wonder of a scented hedgerow in her poem 'The Honeysuckle Fairy' and Thomas Hardy writes about an encounter with a song thrush in 'The Darkling Thrush'. If you prefer paintings, it's worth seeking out the work of artists such as Thomas Gainsborough, JMW Turner and John Ruskin to see the impact such scenes had on them.

UNDERSTANDING THE PURPOSE AND HISTORY OF THE HEDGEROW

In days gone by, hedgerows were managed by hand by skilled practitioners who worked to create a natural boundary made up of tree species that could be shaped by skilful cutting, as well as the occasional large tree specimen like oak or ash. The latter were probably seeded by the birds nesting in the hedge and the skilled hedge layers knew to leave those seedlings to mature and create more height and habitats.

When out walking, check the landscape and you can spot the older hedgerows punctuated by these majestic trees, which were just left to grow. Sometimes, you might come across a row of trees but *no* hedge in fields that have been opened up to allow for larger machinery and higher crop yields. Now you know the story, so you can begin to understand the landscape you are walking through.

Sadly, these days, hedges are often mechanically cut so those precious bird-sown tree saplings are likely to be pruned and never reach maturity. This makes hedges tidy and uniform but, hey, it's better than a fence!

EXPLORING YOUR SENSE OF TASTE: HEDGEROW TEAS AND MORE

Taste is a valuable sense and the simple act of foraging what is currently in season is grounding and rewarding, as every blackberry picker knows. But did you know a typical hedgerow is full of delicious, nutritious and edible plants? In medieval times, hawthorn – a staple hedgerow plant – was even known as 'bread and cheese' because it provided both leaves and flowers to eat. Nettles and cleavers (also known as 'sticky weed' or 'sticky willie' as it clings to clothing – great for sticking on your fellow walkers' backs) that grow at the base of hedges are also full of vital nutrients. To whet your appetite, I have included a few recipes and ideas later in the book (see page 195).

I think the best way to use these plants when walking is to make refreshing teas. Of course, you can pick, dry and store these delights, but there's nothing quite like plucking something fresh, natural and seasonal, and stopping for a brew when you are out for a walk. All you need is a flask of hot water and the knowledge of what is delicious and ripe for picking (see Chapter 8 for information on infuser flasks).

> **TIP**
>
> Nettle seeds can be dried to add to salads, but you will need to learn how to identify male and female ones first. The sparser male seeds won't harm you, but it's the female seeds, which are shaped like little tiny shields and occur in larger, drooping bunches, you want, because they contain the nutritional value.

Look out for these typical hedgerow species to pick and steep for a few minutes for a tasty tea:

- Hawthorn flowers and leaves
- Bramble or blackberry leaves (be careful of thorns) – the leaves were used extensively to replace tea when it was scarce during the wars
- Nettles (you will need gloves but it's worth it) – either fresh or dried
- Cleavers – this plant makes a delicious cold drink with cucumber, too, especially if steeped overnight
- Dandelion flowers and leaves – again fresh or dried will work, but never use the stems as the sap inside is not good

Dos and don'ts for hedgerow foraging

Do:

- Take only what you need, leaving no damage
- Research before trying anything if you have allergies
- Make sure you are 100 per cent sure of any plant you pick – use a plant app or foraging book

Don't:

- Pick anything at dog height
- Pick anything without the landowner's permission (this is illegal, but I generally find picking a few leaves for tea is not frowned upon)
- Mass forage – this strips plants' ability to carry on flowering and producing seeds, and it's sadly on the rise, as anyone who lives near a wild garlic patch will know

'Take the breath of the new dawn and make it part of you. It will give you strength' - Hopi

CASE STUDY: SAM ARMSTRONG

This powerful testimonial from Sam Armstrong outlines the power of walking in nature and connecting with others – the essence of this book.

'Over a decade of caring for my chronically disabled daughter, who underwent pioneering surgery, walking became my lifeline. Each day, I would take a walk while I could, knowing that it would clear my head, release vital endorphins, and give me the strength to face whatever lay ahead. In the midst of an isolated world of caring for a sick child, where the demands were stressful and exhausting, walking allowed me to recharge, focus and find the mental clarity needed to navigate each situation. It became more than just exercise: it was my way of coping, healing and staying strong for my daughter.'

I hope I've shown you how much you can get out of something as simple as walking along a hedgerow. I've experienced the rewards of being immersed in nature myself and I've seen countless other people benefit as well – sometimes their reactions are surprising, sometimes even life-changing – so I hope the practices I've invited you to try here will help *you* make and strengthen your connection to nature, too.

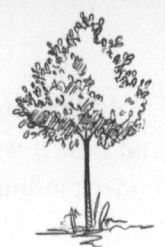

CHAPTER **4**

WALK THIS WAY...
For all-round fitness

Exercise is not complex. There may be a myriad of theories and techniques, but the movements outlined by the original yoga masters or studied by Hippocrates and Michelangelo are essentially the same as those performed by the latest influencers on TikTok – all are based on an understanding of how each muscle works and how to work or stretch it.

To exercise effectively and give your body what it needs for fitness and health, you need to mix up the *types* of exercise you include every week, and I break these down into what I call the three elements of fitness:

1 Cardiovascular (CV) fitness
2 Strength and tone
3 Balance, flexibility and range of movement

Walking for fitness is not about increasing speed or pumping the arms more; it's about understanding these key elements of fitness that our body needs to function well and incorporating them into our walks. While many people stick to just the one element of fitness that they enjoy, you need to include each of these three elements of fitness in order to truly be fit.

Rule number one is that you should always focus on how exercise makes you *feel* rather than how it makes you look. That's because your brain, heart and lungs are as important as your muscles, so read on for a holistic approach to working out that can be incorporated in a walk.

In this chapter, we cover the theory behind each element of fitness and how it will benefit your body. My aim is to arm you with a basic understanding of movement and what to include in your walks to give you all-round fitness and health benefits (see Chapter 5 for exercises and simple fitness walking sequences that build on this knowledge).

Finding a balance

It is common for people to concentrate on either CV exercise like running, cycling or swimming, or more resistance-based strength-and-tone exercise such as weights, body pump or CrossFit – generally, because it's just what they prefer to do.

In the days when I was gym based, I noticed that runners tended to love the treadmills and CV stations, but were less inclined to do weights – perhaps because of the perception that improved muscle tissue might add weight and slow them down – gym-lovers were not so keen to use the treadmills.

That meant even keen exercisers were probably not including all three elements of fitness in their regimes, but we do a balance of all three for true all-round fitness.

Element 1: Cardiovascular (CV) fitness

Put simply, CV means exercise that uses major muscles and is repeated for a sustained period, so you breathe heavily and begin to sweat. The continued use of these muscles requires the heart to pump faster to supply oxygen via the blood and the cellular process, which provides continued energy to the muscles.

CV has huge benefits in relation to metabolism and heart and lung health, but also improves mood, aids sleep, increases energy levels and facilitates weight loss. It differs from strength exercise (see page 60) in that it should elevate the heart rate to at least 50 per cent above its resting levels, ideally for at least 10 minutes.

There are four effective ways to increase the cardiovascular element of a walk:

1 Increase walking speed

2 Use hills, steps and terrain to increase the toughness of a walk

3 Add dynamic moves

4 Use poles to increase the number of major muscles used

In this section we will look at each of these in more detail to help you understand the importance and basics of this 'element'.

How much CV exercise do we need?

Guidelines from the World Health Organization (WHO) and most governments in relation to this type of exercise state that adults should do 150 minutes of moderate-intensity exercise or 75 minutes of more vigorous exercise every week.

The key is to understand what currently constitutes CV exercise for you. It could be walking fast, climbing a hill or running several miles. Next, think about the duration of this exercise and, if you're doing less exercise than the guidelines recommend, aim to gradually increase it.

There are measurements for exercise intensity, such as heart rate monitoring, but if you want to keep things simple, just make sure you regularly push yourself harder. The section on total body walking paces (see page 53) explains how to use intervals and gives you a unique scale to help you recognise when you're increasing the CV element of your walking.

1. Increasing walking speed

It is important to appreciate that simply striving to go faster is not the most effective way to boost CV as you will just become a fast walker with no real way to keep on improving. The key to make walking work is to *alter the pace* to provide different exercise benefits and boost the metabolism.

We'll first explore the many benefits that a 'brisk' pace can offer – and why mixing it up can be more effective than typical high-intensity interval training (HIIT) circuit workouts. Then, at the end of the section, I'll explain why *slow* can be good, too.

THE BENEFITS OF 'BRISK'

Brisk walking has been the subject of many research projects, healthy-living guidelines and magazine articles in recent years, especially in relation to brain function, heart health, ageing and longevity. For example, to mention just one, a 2017 report by Harvard Health found that walking briskly for 20 minutes a day could reduce the risk of heart disease by up to 30 per cent.

Brisk walking may also slow the ageing process. Telomeres are part of our DNA and sit at the end of chromosomes to stop them getting damaged. They tend to shorten as we age, so longer telomeres are associated with longer life expectancy. A 2022 study published by Leicester University found that, when their DNA was studied, those who self-reported as being brisk walkers typically had longer telomeres and therefore were likely to live longer. Similarly, a 2017 study published in science journal *PeerJ* looked at the relationship between brisk walking and dementia in healthy older adults. They found that adults who went on regular brisk walks performed cognitive tasks better than adults who did not walk regularly.

The evidence for the benefits of brisk walking is strong, but how do you work out what a brisk walk is and, more importantly, how do you deploy this secret walking weapon?

WHAT IS A BRISK PACE?

This is one of those 'how long is a piece of string' questions, because obviously it depends on bodyweight, age, health, the terrain you are walking over and a myriad of other factors. 'Brisk' also means different things to different individuals – for one it could be very gentle while for another it could mean maximum speed. For the general population (average adult walkers) two reliable measures that tend to be used depending on how you might wish to track your pace are:

- Steps per minute – use a step counter app or fitness tracker – around 100 steps per minute is brisk for an average adult.
- Miles per hour – this is the measure used in the NHS Active 10 tracker app (see page 144) – approximately 3–3.5 miles per hour is brisk for an average adult.

If you are a naturally fast walker, you may want to focus on both steps per minute *and* miles per hour, but if walking for a set amount of time is too challenging (or too difficult to measure), you may initially find it easier to focus on steps per minute.

A more natural way to determine walking pace is by how it makes you *feel*. If the two measures above aren't helpful to you or you prefer not to use trackers, focus on how you feel using the total body walking pace scale below. This works best if you understand how you move naturally while walking (see Chapter 1), because then you will understand the effort levels and can maintain a good walking technique for posture and comfort.

TOTAL BODY WALKING PACES

There are three paces, determined by how a walk feels and the effort required. Simple cues will teach you how to monitor your pace, and use it to get the most out of your walks. Here is how to work out your own levels using a simple 1 to 10 intensity scale.

POSTURAL PACE (PACE 1)

This is a gentle pace where you have a relaxed posture and don't feel you're making *too* much effort. You should be able to chat, and feel in control of your breathing and flowing movements. Effort level: 3/10.

PURPOSEFUL PACE (PACE 2)

Here you up the ante a bit and begin to add more *purpose* to the pace, with increased body movement such as arm swing. This will mean your breathing will be slightly heavier, but you should still be able to say a sentence, although it will be more strained, with maybe a gap or two for breath. You will be 'glowing' a bit too. You should be able to comfortably hold your posture and a good walking style. Effort level: 5/10.

PERFORMANCE PACE (PACE 3)

Talking should now be a couple of words between breaths and you will be 'hotting up' and breaking into a sweat. There should be an increased range of movement in both stride and arm swing (or pole technique) and you will be moving faster. Avoid the temptation to pump the arms and lose good posture, as this will result in smaller steps. This pace is ideal for intervals, as the idea is to get the heart pumping fast. Effort level: 9/10.

Note: Trying to walk too fast without practice is likely to cause shin pain, because your leg muscles are not used to keeping your toes up and rolling through the foot. Often confused with shin splints, this results in a burning pain which can ease when you stop, but will become acute if you do not build up gradually and take time to stretch after your walk.

A simple rule of thumb is: if it is uncomfortable, peg it back. You want to build your fitness and enjoy walking, not injure yourself by doing too much too soon.

RECOVERY PACE

It is important not to ignore how beneficial slow walking can be for your health, so don't base everything around speed. Every burst of speed should be accompanied by a rest period. In this section we use a rest and recovery process, which will improve our performance on each repetition of an exercise. Walking slowly is also proven to improve brain function and concentration (see Chapter 2 for how it can benefit mental health).

Understanding HIIT

HIIT is a popular way to boost cardiovascular fitness and is more effective than pushing yourself over a sustained period. In short, you use condensed bursts of very high intensity accompanied by rest periods. You may have heard of HIIT circuits, which became very popular in the last decade, but the principle has been used by runners for far longer. It's mainly known as fartlek training (it means 'speed play' in Swedish and was devised by an Olympian).

The benefits of HIIT:

- It improves cardiovascular fitness more quickly than same-pace walking.
- It is quick to do, so is great if you are time limited.
- It builds endurance and trains the body to utilise its energy systems effectively.
- If you can maintain the bursts for at least 30–60 seconds at a time, you'll get an endorphin kick too.

54 WALK THIS WAY

2. Using hills, steps and terrain to increase the toughness of a walk

If the terrain you're walking on makes your walk tougher, it will add to the training effect. That might be uneven ground, soft sinking sand or slippery mud. All are great reasons to walk outdoors and challenge your body in different ways. In most areas, the greatest natural CV trainer will be hills. Just incorporating an incline into your route – or at least not avoiding them – will provide a fitness bonus.

Here's why hills are so good for us:

- They increase exercise intensity and calories burned (this increases by gradient).
- They activate the lower leg muscles – great for strengthening ankles.
- They target different upper leg muscles – specifically hamstrings and glutes.
- They prepare you for tougher terrain.

HOW DO YOU MEASURE A GRADIENT?

On roads, there are signs showing significant gradients, but this information is only really made available for walkers via specific walking routes and typically only in the wilder hilly areas. The best way to check out how hilly a route is or the gradient of a walk you have completed is via apps such as MapMyWalk (see page 144).

HOW TO CLIMB AND DESCEND HILLS

To save your knees from too much strain, here are a few tips to help you walk with good posture and awareness both up and down hills:

UPHILL

- Do not lean into a hill – keep your centre of gravity upright where possible.
- Use poles to spread the load – you may need to shorten them.
- Maintain a steady pace and minimise stops – slow and steady with a good rhythm is better than bursts with a break, as that loses momentum.

- Mix up your steps – longer, shorter – to challenge different muscles.
- On tough climbs, some hill walkers also straighten their back leg and pause every now and then, thus taking the strain off the muscles.

DOWNHILL

- Maintain your centre of gravity by keeping your body nice and low, but over your legs. Don't lean too far backwards or forwards.
- Lengthen your poles, if you are using them.
- Zigzag along a path to avoid too much weight going through your knees and shins.
- Turn sideways on to a drop – your knees will thank you for it.
- Shorten your stride, even if it feels counterintuitive.
- Try to keep your lead leg semi-bent when it hits the ground to reduce impact on your joints.

For some great ideas for using hills and steps to boost CV training, see page 75.

3. Adding dynamic moves

Technically, these fall into another category called plyometric exercises, but they are also great for increasing the heart rate, so I will include them in this section.

SKIPPING

Literally replicating that joyful movement children do, skipping has a similar effect to a fast burst of exercise and it works on coordination and balance too. Start with a low skipping action. Take it slowly to begin with, and gradually aim to go higher and travel further with each skip. Only a few skips are needed and you can add them anywhere in a walk, as long as you have warmed up.

HOPPING

Hopping has similar benefits to skipping, but as you put all your weight on to one leg, be careful and start gently. The hops also provide bone-strengthening benefits. You can hop from one leg to the other or do a series of hops per leg. Build up as you get more confident and proficient.

BOUNDING

This is a more advanced action that is almost a combination of skipping and hopping. Start off as if you are skipping, but then push off harder with one leg and take your opposite knee higher. As you bounce up, you should bend the arm opposite to that raised knee at 90 degrees (square), while keeping the other arm straight by your side. Alternate this pattern, making sure you stop if you lose form (see the puppet master sequence on page 96 for ideas that use a similar move).

JUMPING

Jumping with two feet can be done on the spot, but when walking I like to keep moving forward, so a small two-footed 'bunny hop' is a great way to challenge your muscles and CV system. Impact is also great for bone strengthening, so give it a go.

4. Using poles to increase the number of major muscles used

There is one way to walk that includes the three elements of fitness in one go, so if you are time poor but want to make walking your workout, pick up a pair of poles. The emphasis is on *pair*. I do not advocate using one pole when walking (unless you have to for mobility reasons), because it is unbalanced and causes a lean to one side and an unnatural spinal position (see page 58 for pole types and adjustments).

THE BENEFITS OF USING POLES

When poles are used properly, the benefits are massive:

- They engage 90 per cent of major muscles, providing a whole-body workout with every step.
- They reduce the pressure on lower-body joints like knees and hips.
- They tone the upper body as well as the legs, but it's vital to avoid short, square-arm movements (see page 84)
- They can increase calorie consumption from 20 to 40 per cent, depending on technique and intensity, and can thus help with weight loss.
- Propulsion makes you lighter on your feet, which makes it possible to walk further and faster than usual.

- They engage the core and improve the posture, natural wrist position and gait.

In short, it's like the difference between using a treadmill and a cross trainer in the gym – except you are outdoors!

TRADITIONAL NORDIC WALKING

Nordic walking originated in Finland, where using two poles to add exercise to walking was first embraced in the 1940s by cross-country skiers who wanted to train in the summer. They replicated the long, flowing movement of skiing and by the 1990s it had become a sport. Used initially to train the army, it soon became apparent that this activity was a great workout that could be done by anyone, anywhere.

I have been involved in the delivery and development of Nordic walking for people of different fitness and ability levels since 2008. Over the years I have tried almost every exercise fad going and it is the most effective way to exercise that I have encountered, but, as I outline in the second edition of my book *The Complete Guide to Nordic Walking*, it is the latest developments in pole walking that excite me the most.

The original Nordic techniques accurately mirrored a quite regimented movement with a lot of dos and don'ts, and while many of us tried to make it more achievable, we did find the average walker often ended up tapping their poles and not getting the full benefits. This was mainly because the action was designed to produce a long stride that matched the glide length of skiing and required the participant to be attached to the poles by glove-like straps, which enabled them to 'push and let go'.

This cannot be achieved with the looped strap commonly found on trekking poles, so specific poles are required. Because the activity requires forward propulsion, it is also necessary to angle the poles, so they are planted into the ground behind the body to aid a pushing forward motion. This action, the correct arm swing and articulation through the straps take a bit of practice and tuition from a trained instructor.

FITNESS POLES

Fitness poles are a more recent innovation. They come with a moulded ergonomic handle that replaces the need for the straps, and are fitted to poles with a shaft that is angled at the top by 15 degrees. Although at first glance they look like most other trekking or hiking poles, the handle is designed to mirror your hand position when you walk without poles – a natural curl with your thumb at the top. This makes them much more 'grab and go', with less opportunity to get things wrong, because once in the hand the poles automatically sit at the correct angle and it is impossible to over-grip them (another common issue with traditional poles).

Walking with fitness poles gives you a much more natural stride and a more relaxed arm movement, yet engages the core and upper body more (see page 78 to master using fitness poles). The design was based on adding power to a natural walking pattern, which also means the wrist is in a neutral position and less likely to feel strained or be injured. When you are not strapped to the poles it also makes it easier to add strength and balance exercises, pick flowers to go in your tea or take your coat on and off. This is why I recommend them if you want to get more out of every step without feeling like you're marching. I see them as the ultimate tool for the walker who wants to enjoy all the benefits outlined in this book.

Walking vs. running as 'proper exercise'

I want to reiterate why I believe walking is the ultimate exercise by comparing it to running, which many might consider 'proper exercise'. Agreed, regular runners will have great cardiovascular fitness and good leg muscles, but unless they also do some other form of exercise they often lack upper-body strength and good posture.

Walking, on the other hand – especially using poles – works out the upper body and core as well as the lower body, enabling us to improve circulation and heart function, strengthen muscles and bones. It also promotes weight loss and improves our posture.

Many runners seem to miss the power of nature as they zoom past and concentrate on their watches. With walking, as we immerse ourselves in the elements of the great outdoors, we can take more time to look around us, have some space for our thoughts and be mindful, which has no end of mental health benefits, reducing the risk of stress, anxiety and depression.

Element 2: Strength and tone

The second element of fitness we will explore is all about keeping muscles strong through what is known as resistance exercise. This is a key factor in maintaining a good quality of life, moving correctly and ageing well. Building it into your total body walking plan (see the Appendix) will increase the value you get from every step.

If our work or daily lives do not involve lifting, pushing, bending and physical labour that requires our muscles to be constantly challenged, they will simply lose strength and mass. Through to our late twenties this is not so noticeable, but the decline in lean tissue begins to show from our thirties onwards and increases year on year. Not only does it affect how we look and feel, but it also rapidly increases our risk of ill health. In later life it is cited as the major risk of falls and hospitalisation.

It is simple to maintain strength without having to go to a gym and it is a myth that exercises that build strength also build bulk. Simply adding some exercises to your walk will make a huge difference. Like everything I advocate, we just need to move the body as nature intended by working the muscles hard enough to cause the fibres to break down and rebuild (which is entirely natural). To do this, we need the muscles to work against some kind of resistance or weight – hence resistance or weight training.

Resistance training can be done with lifting, pushing or pulling actions, which make the muscles work as fully as possible, either individually or as a group. Resistance can be achieved by using bodyweight – as in a press-up – or with a weighted object, band or similar that makes the action harder. The idea is to repeat the action a few times, possibly with a short rest in between every 10 repetitions or so.

Note: The terms 'repetitions' (or 'reps') and 'sets' are widely used when people talk about strength exercises. Repetitions means the number of times you repeat the exercise and sets are the number of times you repeat that number.

In the next chapter, you will find a few well-known exercises that work a couple of muscle groups together and are easy to perform without too much equipment (see page 85). These are the basis for my simple walking-based sequences, which are as multifunctional as possible.

The benefits of strength exercise

Resistance exercise:

- Improves the ability to perform everyday tasks with ease and comfort.
- Helps maintain a healthy weight by increasing calorie consumption.
- Improves muscle tone.
- Improves heart health.
- Reduces the risk of falls.
- Aids the management of blood sugar levels.
- Boosts brain health.

TIP

Performing more exercises with a manageable weight is the most effective way to trigger these benefits, so avoid the temptation to strain against heavy resistance and aim for endurance instead – far easier to do en route!

How does building more lean tissue help with weight loss?

Put simply, when we ask the muscles to work against resistance, they require energy. Fat that is stored in the muscles, liver and tissue is broken down by the muscles with the help of oxygen to provide that energy. To gain the oxygen, we need to breathe harder, meaning that resistance exercise has an element of CV too.

After you have finished a walk involving strength exercises, your oxygen uptake remains elevated to restore your muscles to their resting state. This phenomenon, known as afterburn (or post-exercise oxygen consumption), elevates our metabolisms. The increased percentage in lean tissue directly increases the calories your body consumes when you are not exercising too. Your body simply becomes a much more efficient 'engine' when at rest or in action.

Strength training works at any age. Simon attended group walks that included strength exercises and noticed a huge difference.

'This is so important, especially for older folk. I am in my seventies and have been working at this for about a year. I feel measurably stronger and fitter for it. It doesn't have to be a boot camp with someone shouting at you. Anything that involves some resistance will help. I can now carry two 15kg (33lb) suitcases up a flight of stairs at an airport rather than having to take the lift. I can lift them into the overhead locker on the plane with no help, too. I would encourage everyone to do some kind of resistance exercise as well as walking. Go for it. You're worth it.'

How frequently do we need to do strength exercises?

The WHO guidelines advise that adults between 19 and 64 should do strengthening activities that work all the major muscle groups – legs, hips, back, stomach, chest, shoulders and arms – at least twice a week. I use these guidelines when I help you create a total body walking plan (see the Appendix), which will help you select the types and quantity of exercises that will build all-round fitness. The key is to perform strength exercises on, as a minimum, two of your walks each week, ideally by including two leg and two upper-body exercises each time, but if you prefer you could do legs one day and arms another day. Once you know how to mix and match your walking moves and daily inspirations (see Chapter 10), you may soon want to do strength exercises more than twice a week, which is fine.

The four basic full-body strength moves

To keep things simple, I have chosen four basic strength exercises that are suitable for building into a total body walking plan:

1 Squat
2 Lunge

3 Chest press
4 Triceps dip

Some involve stepping and moving, while others can be done at intervals on a daily walk. All will help to tone muscles, boost metabolism and build strength. You can find out how to perform these safely on page 85.

If you like to keep things simple, you can just memorise the basic format and build progression by simply doing more. If you want to add variety and challenge your body in more ways, choose from the variations and fitness walking sequences on page 94.

Element 3: Balance, flexibility and range of movement

This is actually a group of elements that work together to improve how you move in everyday life, but they are closely interlinked, so to keep things simple I have put them together. They all relate to using our bodies effectively, and are the basis for good posture and understanding our natural movement while walking.

As you work through this book, you will see how they appear in the fitness walking sequences (see page 94) and how you can add them into your daily walks. You will soon notice that you walk more efficiently, feel better and ward off or reduce aches and pains both when walking and when performing everyday tasks.

Let's explore each one in turn to understand why they appear in all of the fitness walking sequences. We'll start with the key one, balance, which requires more practice than the others.

Balance

Often overlooked, balance is something that declines quickly but can be improved at any age. It is a vital component in everything, from the ability to stand up straight to our reactions and range of movement. I often find people are not interested in this until it matters, but working on balance suddenly makes a myriad of movements feel smoother and more comfortable. I urge you to give my basic balance moves (see page 91) a go. I have seen massive improvements in people who thought they were fit and certainly never knew they needed to improve their balance.

It is vital to take a holistic approach to all movement. All-round fitness includes the links between our eyes, brain, vestibular system (the sensory organs in the inner ear) and joints – they *all* work together to keep us upright and mobile, and *all* need stimulation and exercising to stay in good condition. Poor function of any one of these systems makes it more difficult to balance and will increase the risk of stumbles and falls.

Balance exercises naturally engage the body's core muscles and help us to correct our body positions quickly to adjust to a shift in weight distribution, such as a misstep off a kerb or walking on uneven ground. A few exercises to activate the core, improve leg and hip strength and practise foot lifts can make a huge difference. For older adults, it can ensure they stay mobile and reduce the risk of falling. As decline begins to become evident in mid-life, it's never too early to start. In fact, up to 45 per cent of falls are known to be due to a balance decline, which sets in much earlier than people think.

Including a few balance exercises in your daily regime will make a huge difference (see page 91 for a range of balance exercises). By simply closing your eyes on some exercises, you remove the signals from your visual system and put greater emphasis on the signals from your vestibular system and the receptors in your joints and muscles (proprioception).

Flexibility

Flexibility is one of the elements that suddenly becomes of interest to people once stiffness creeps in. Again, unless it's due to not stretching properly after strenuous exercise, this happens earlier than people might imagine. Either way, nobody wants to be the one who groans when picking something up or getting off the sofa, so understanding how to stay flexible is a valuable tool. It also prevents muscle injuries and joint problems, and improves overall performance.

There is no need for specific flexibility practice as just performing the cool-down stretches on page 72 will help enormously. The yoga moves in Chapter 2 and the fitness walking sequences on page 94 also contain ways to improve flexibility.

Range of movement – functional fitness

Interlinked with flexibility and strength, range of movement refers to the ability of your muscles and joints to function to their full potential. Functional fitness means the ability to perform daily movements such as bending, twisting, lifting, pulling and pushing.

If we do not perform such moves, we simply lose the ability to do them with ease. If you know what to do and how good it can feel once you have mastered it, your reward is a body with joints that are kept loose and muscles that work as they are intended to in everyday life. For me, exercise should ideally make everyday living easier and movement a joy. With the fitness walking sequences I have put together (see page 94), you will see how you can 'layer' the elements to improve all-round fitness and mobility.

Once again, there is no need to practise, but if you do incorporate the fitness walking sequences into your walks, you will notice that they encourage these vital movements.

AGILITY

Agility exercises are not something you might associate with an exercise regime for general well-being, as they are typically used for sports coaching, yet being able to move quickly and change direction can help you cope with the unexpected (dog, car, cyclist, rabbit hole, raised paving stones, for example) or when walking on difficult terrain, especially when going downhill.

I love to include some faster light footwork in a total body walking plan (see the Appendix). These small, fast moves, with added changes in direction, are brilliant for training our body to be able to react and move quickly when we need to. Simply stepping on the spot with fast feet and soft knees is a good way to start – keeping your feet closer to the ground than when performing balance exercises. Once you get used to these faster bursts of footwork, start using them when travelling forwards too.

IMPACT

You will note that in some fitness walking sequences (see page 94), I include a bouncing or jumping action. This is to build in some impact with the ground, as this is what helps to keep our bones strong, and jumping moves also boost CV, strength, balance and good posture. The Royal Osteoporosis Society advises that everyone – even those with osteoporosis – incorporates 50 moderate impacts (jumps, skips, jogs or hops) on most days.

Coupled with resistance exercise, adding a few impact or weight-bearing exercises to a walk will stimulate the renewal of bone cells, leading to denser, stronger bones. It doesn't matter if you're young or old, overweight or in great shape, learn a few moves, but *never* attempt them until you are fully warmed up.

POSTURE

However, as I outlined in Chapter 1, good posture is the foundation for all the other elements. If you build any of them around poor posture, you will limit their effectiveness and can even cause injury in the longer term. Remember that good posture enables efficient movement and good breathing, and that sitting plays havoc with our postural muscles. As well as walking daily, using poles and working on the three elements of fitness, take a break from sitting every 40 minutes or so or choose a desk that allows to you to work in a standing position.

Now we've covered the theory behind the three elements of fitness and why they're important, let's move on to some practical exercises you can try while you're out walking that incorporate those elements.

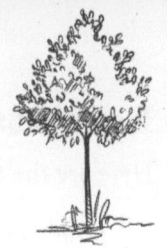

CHAPTER

5

WALK THIS WAY...
For practical exercises and fitness walking sequences

This chapter is full of easy-to-follow exercises to boost your fitness as you walk, listed in order of the element of fitness they target most. These are followed by some fitness walking sequences (see page 94), which include a good mix of all three elements of fitness.

But first you need to understand how to prepare your body for walking and increasing your activity levels. As with any exercise, you need to warm up and afterwards you need to cool down. The result? You will look forward to your walks and gain something positive from every step.

The warm-up and cool-down

It's a great idea to get into the habit of preparing your body before a walk and thanking it afterwards with a lovely stretch. Allowing the body to warm up gradually and settle back after exertion will prevent soreness and injury, and make you move and feel better.

Benefits of a warm-up

Here are the benefits of doing a warm-up sequence:

- It increases the temperature within the muscles used – once warmed up, a muscle can contract more forcefully and relax more quickly.
- It decreases the risk of injury – a warm muscle is less likely to be overstretched and will be less prone to injury.
- The blood vessels will dilate – this reduces resistance to blood flow and lowers stresses on the heart.
- It increases blood temperature – as blood travels through the muscles its temperature rises and its haemoglobin (the protein in red blood cells) releases oxygen more readily. This can enhance endurance.
- It improves the range of joint motion – for most of us, the ability to move our joints freely and comfortably, especially when walking faster or on uneven ground, is one of the most important benefits of warming up.
- It causes hormonal changes – your body increases its production of various hormones responsible for regulating energy production when you are active. During warm-up, the balance of hormones responsible for regulating energy production makes more carbohydrates and fatty acids available.
- It prepares you mentally – a warm-up allows you time to relax and prepare mentally for your walk, and whether it's mindful or a full-blown workout walk, it will enable you to focus more on what you want to gain.

How to warm up

The best way to approach a warm-up is to think of the joints you will be using and take them through some simple mobilisation exercises. These should always relate to the actions required in the activity you are about to undertake (in this case, walking). If you have already completed the checks in Chapter 1, you should be familiar with many of these movements already and will not need to memorise lots of new ones.

Why warm up?

Joints contain synovial fluid, which lubricates them, nourishes the surrounding tissues and helps with shock absorption. When you have been static for a while, it settles and becomes less viscous, so these joint movements are great at any time and really do aid mobility.

Full-body warm-up sequence

THE OPTIMUM WARM-UP STANCE

When warming up, start from the feet up and assume this body position:

- Stand upright with good alignment of your head, ribcage and pelvis.
- Draw your abdominals gently in towards your spine to stabilise your pelvis, keeping it still during the exercise.
- Plant your feet hip-width apart for balance.
- Keep your knees 'soft' when standing. When bending your knees, your weight should be back so that your knees don't travel in front of the feet. Your knees should remain in line with your second and third toes.

> **TIP**
>
> While the optimum warm-up stance is desirable, some people do not have the physical make-up to allow this to be achieved. In such instances, limit the range of movement so that your joint and limb positions are maintained.

WARMING UP BEFORE A WALK

These moves should only be done 6–10 times, so your warm-up should be complete in under 10 minutes. You will notice that as you proceed through this sequence you gradually add more muscle actions as well as joint mobilisation. This is to slowly increase the blood flow and heart rate.

1 **Ankle rotations** – Simply stand on one leg (which is great for balance, but if you need to, hold on to something). Rotate the ankle on the lifted leg in one direction, before repeating in the other direction. Next point the toes up and down a few times. Repeat with the other leg.

2 **Foot rolls** – These simply imitate the movement we do when planting our feet. Stand on one leg and place the heel of the other leg on the ground so you can roll through the sole of the foot and up on to the toes. Either repeat 8–10 times on this foot before switching or alternate with the other foot, which is more like actual walking.

3 **Knee lifts** – Lift one leg at a time to march on the spot, taking your knees to hip height if you can.

4 **Buttock kicks** – Kick one leg at a time behind you, taking your foot as close to your buttocks as it will go. As you step from leg to leg, switch the weight from side to side to make the move more dynamic.

5 **Hip swings** – Stand on one leg and, without being aggressive, swing the lifted leg forwards and backwards to mobilise the hip joint. Next, take the leg across the body to just past the centre point, before taking it out to the side slightly. Repeat with the other leg.

6 **Waist bends** – Stand facing forward, keeping your pelvis still, and place your hands on the side of your thighs. Bend gently to the side, sliding your hand towards your knee, first one side and then the other. This mobilises the spine, so be careful not to overdo it. To add some intensity, you could raise the hand that is not sliding down towards your head.

7 **Spinal rotations** – Start gently by keeping your feet on the ground while taking both arms out to the sides, just below shoulder height. Without tensing your shoulders, gently rotate your arms from side to side. To increase intensity, you can begin to swing more vigorously and start stepping across from side to side as you go. This is great for preparing your back before a walk.

8 **Shoulder swim** – Standing tall, begin to 'swim' forwards, making a reaching motion with your arms, as if doing front crawl. Make sure you reach back before pulling your arm forward again. As you do this large arm movement, notice how your trunk rotates. Then reverse the movement so you are swimming backwards (as long as

your shoulders are comfortable with that). You could do both arms together to reach forward and then take them out to the sides as if performing a breast stroke, too.

TIP

You can warm up indoors and be more static, but if you are outdoors it is always good to be as dynamic as possible to avoid getting chilly.

Benefits of a cool-down

After a walk – even a gentle one – it's essential to gently cool your muscles down and stretch them out, rather than stopping suddenly and jumping into the car or sitting back down. Muscles are made up of masses of fibres that contract and shorten when worked hard, so it's important to lengthen them after using them for a 'workout' (whatever the level of exertion) to help them to recover from the activity, and improve their condition and tone, rather than allowing them to simply tighten and feel sore. Stretching also conditions the tendons that connect the muscles to your bones, so regular gentle stretching gradually improves your range of movement – and it feels good, too.

Doing a cool-down sequence:

- Improves range of motion
- Decreases joint stiffness
- Decreases muscle tension
- Improves posture
- Improves circulation
- Provides time to relax

How to cool down

Towards the end of a more vigorous walk, make a conscious decision to ease back on your pace and effort/intensity. Allow your heart rate to slow before assuming the same position as for the optimum warm-up (see page 69).

Try to lightly engage the abdominals at all times and to maintain a straight back while stretching, particularly when holding a stretch involving a forward bend, such as a hamstring stretch.

Full-body cool-down routine

Relax and breathe normally while working through the stretches, and *never* rush them or hold for a few seconds only. Stretching is something to enjoy and take your time over. For maximum effect, every movement should be held for 10–30 seconds. You will soon notice that your ability to stretch further will increase over time.

Never 'bounce' or force a stretch – the movement should be gradual. Remember to stretch to the point of tension – never push through pain – and do not perform these stretches on cold muscles. Have a structured stretch routine to avoid imbalances between areas of your body.

1 **Calves** – Stand upright and take a good step back with one leg, while bending the front leg to aid this movement. Retain good posture and make sure the rear heel is on the ground, not lifted. Check that the bent knee does not go past the toes and both feet are front facing. You should feel a lovely stretch in the calf muscle of the rear leg. Hold and breathe smoothly, then repeat with the other leg.

2 **Hamstrings (back of thighs)** – Stand upright and then bend both legs slightly, keeping them close together with the hands on the front of the thighs, before kicking one leg forward so the heel is on the ground. Bend slightly over that leg, while keeping the hands on the thighs to protect your back. You may want to point the toes away from or towards you. Do what is comfortable but check that you are feeling the stretch in your hamstrings.

3 **Quadriceps (front of thighs)** – Stand and raise the heel of one leg behind you as if you were aiming to touch your backside with your foot. If you can, use the hand on the same side to hold the foot (or grab your trousers or socks, if it helps) in that position until you feel a stretch across the front of the thigh. Keep the other hand free in case you need to hold on to something. Hold the foot in this

position for 10–30 seconds before releasing and repeating on the other side. If this is too tough, you can find a bench to rest the front of the foot on in a similar position. You may need to bend the knee of the standing leg to feel the stretch in the front of the leg with the foot on the bench.

4 **Waist stretch** – For this stretch, repeat the warm-up waist bends (see page 70), but always add the raised arm and move slowly, holding the bent position.

5 **Back stretch** – Bend over with your hands on your thighs and knees slightly bent, keeping your back flat and using your hands to take the weight of your upper body. Gently arch the centre of your back upwards and then reverse this by arching it downwards. (If you have ever seen the yoga Cat and Cow poses, you will know what I mean.)

6 **Chest stretch** – Stand straight and interlock your hands behind your back before lifting them away from your body, taking them upwards slightly, if you can. It is important to breathe deeply to lift the breastbone and keep your core engaged so you do not overarch your back. Hold for 10–30 seconds to feel the stretch before relaxing and releasing the fingers.

7 **Upper back and shoulders** – Stand straight and take one arm across the body at shoulder height, making sure there is space between it and your body before holding it in the opposite hand, just above the elbow. Make sure your shoulder stays down and is not tensed or raised. Use the gripping hand to gently pull the arm towards the opposite side, creating a stretch across the upper back. Breathe between your shoulder blades to feel the stretch as you hold. Gently release and repeat on the other side.

8 **Triceps stretch (backs of the arms)** – Stand straight and take one arm upwards close to your ear on the same side. Bend that arm backwards so your hand is reaching down towards your shoulder, while holding it in position with the opposite hand on the back of your upper arm. To stretch, use this hand to either hold the arm in place or, if you can manage it, push it back slightly. Hold this stretch before releasing your arm and repeating on the other side.

These warm-up and cool-down exercises will soon become second nature as you begin to enjoy them without having to think about them.

Now that we know how to warm up and cool down, I will run through some exercises for each of the three elements of fitness. You can approach these exercises in two ways: with a pick 'n' mix approach, where you casually pick out any exercise you feel like doing, or by selecting a range of exercises to incorporate into your total body walking plan (see the Appendix), should you choose to create one.

Element 1: Cardiovascular exercises

Pace/speed intervals

Here is a simple 30-minute plan for varying the pace of your walking in intervals, using the paces on page 53 to make it simpler. Perform the warm-up sequence on page 69 before starting to alternate between performance and purposeful pace. Do not begin faster paces until you have walked for a few minutes to prepare the body. Follow the table below. The performance pace comes in 2-minute bursts, which should be as fast as possible, while maintaining good form. See page 54 for more detailed information about interval training.

If a 30-minute session is not achievable for you, break the exercise down to 10 minutes, starting with the first 10 minutes in the table and adding a cool-down at the end. Gradually add more time as you understand what your body is comfortable doing.

Note: This does not have to be a specific fitness walk as the principle can be used on any walk – just up the ante for a couple of minutes and drop back down to a resting pace. You will manage longer bursts of intensity as you get fitter – and will notice the results, too.

Minutes	Pace
0–3	Warm-up — **moderate** pace
5–7	**Performance** pace
7–8	**Purposeful** pace
8–10	**Performance** pace
10–11	**Purposeful** pace
11–13	**Performance** pace
13–14	**Purposeful** pace

14–16	**Performance** pace
16–17	**Purposeful** pace
17–19	**Performance** pace
19–20	**Purposeful** pace
20–22	**Performance** pace
22–23	**Purposeful** pace
23–25	**Performance** pace
25–30	Cool-down

Hills

Here are two hillwalking exercises to boost your CV workouts. See page 55 for more detailed information and hill techniques.

1. HILLWALKING VARIATION EXERCISES

Even a small slope can be a great workout opportunity. Some simple variations for hillwalking are:

- Climb up the hill slowly and descend quickly.
- Climb up the hill quickly and descend slowly as a rest period.
- Turn sideways on the steps and take 10 steps up the hill with the leg that faces them. Turn to the other side and take another 10 steps up the hill. Then come down normally.
- Walk backwards uphill and come down frontwards.
- Make wide zigzags up a slope so you are walking from side to side on the hill rather than going up in a straight line. This increases the time climbing, but reduces the impact of the gradient.
- Zigzag downhill to ease your knees.

2. THE EVEREST CLIMB

This is a version of a 'never-ending hill climb', which you can adapt accordingly. It is my favourite way of turning a hill into a great workout.

- On the first ascent, mark out four 'stations' using anything bright. I call these my camps: 'Base Camp', 'Camp 1', 'Camp 2' and 'Camp 3'.
- On the second ascent, walk to Base Camp and back down to the start before climbing up again, passing all camps and getting to the summit. Now go back to the start.

- On the third ascent, walk to Camp 2 and back to Base Camp, before climbing up again, passing all camps and getting to the summit. Go back to the start.
- On the fourth ascent, walk to Camp 3, drop down to Camp 2 before climbing up again, passing all camps and getting to the summit. Go back to the start.

TIP

If hills hurt your knees – use poles (see page 57).

'To climb steep hills requires a slow pace at first' – William Shakespeare

Step aerobics

One of the simplest ways to add more intensity to a walk is to find a flight of steps, which could be a road or railway bridge, a bandstand in a park, or rugged steps cut into a wilder natural hill. You can even do these exercises indoors – office buildings with several flights are ideal.

What follows are five simple step aerobic exercises that you can use by either building all five into a comprehensive workout or simply boost your daily walk by adding just one of these to the steps you pass. Progress by increasing the number of repetitions or doing a circuit of all five before repeating them.

Try to locate suitable steps on your usual routes (ideally equal in step height, with at least 10 of them). Once you get competent at these exercises, you will be able to drop them in to any walk where you happen upon a suitable flight of stairs. Bear in mind that steps can vary in depth and may be wide, narrow or uneven – use this variety as much as you can to challenge your body and boost your CV workout. As well as giving you increased CV intensity, you will notice that this step aerobics programme also incorporates the other three elements of fitness.

Of course, it is important your muscles are warm before increasing your activity levels to this intensity, so make sure you warm up before beginning (see page 69).

1. SIDE STEPS

- Stand side-on at the base of the steps, with one leg facing the steps and the other away from them.
- With the leg closest to the steps remaining facing to the side, begin to climb them one at a time. This works the muscles in a totally different way to walking, and you will need to take it easy to start with. Try to climb at least 10 steps before stepping back down again using the *same* leg.
- Once at the bottom, turn to face the other way, with the leg that just did all the work facing *away* from the steps. Repeat the action with the second leg.

2. DOUBLE-UPS

For this exercise, you will need steps that are not too deep.

- Step up two steps at a time. Do this steadily, then come down as fast as you can, using every step.
- Repeat this process of deep steps up and small, faster steps down as many times as you can manage. Aim to build up to 10 sets.

3. BALANCE STEPS

- For this exercise, bend your knee as if to take each step, but before placing your foot down, pause and remain with it lifted for the count of five.
- Place it down and repeat with the other leg. Once you reach the top, come back down quickly and repeat.

4. NEVER-ENDING STEPS

This exercise really makes a flight of steps hard work, so it is great even if you can only manage a few steps.

- Climb two of the steps, taking each one separately, and then step back down one while still facing the steps. Next take another two steps, one at a time, and repeat the step back down, and so on.

- Once at the top, come down quickly and repeat.
- You could alter this to take one large step down that takes in two steps at the same time.

5. SKATER STEPS

In this exercise you are stepping out to each side like a skater. It's a great way to work the outer and inner thighs, and an action that we do not often manage.

- Take a wide a step to the right with the right leg and repeat with the left.
- When you reach the top, come back down with normal steps before repeating.
- The number of repetitions depends on the numbers of steps available.

Using fitness poles

Once you master walking with fitness poles, you will be able to do it anywhere. Just 20 minutes a day will make a huge difference, and the action can be adjusted to suit your particular body, fitness levels and goals. I frequently meet people who simply can't believe the results they are getting from using them. For more information on using fitness poles, see page 81.

On a safety note, I always advise users of strapped poles to unclip them on tricky terrain or before descending a steep path, so your hands are free to break any fall and because, if you're 'strapped in' and fall, it can result in thumb injuries. For the same reason, I do not advise those with balance conditions to be strapped into any poles at any time. Similarly, to fully experience the benefits, freedom and natural workout of total body walking, a light grip on ergonomic handles is preferable.

HOW TO HOLD AND USE FITNESS POLES

STEP 1

Notice how, when you swing your arm from the shoulder in a more 'triangular' movement (rather than pumping the arms with a bend at the elbow), your hand is naturally loosely curled with your thumb at the top.

STEP 2

- Make sure you are holding the ergonomic handles correctly and that they are in the right hands. Each will have a small ledge at the base and a thumb ridge that assists you to mirror the natural hand position above.
- Place the edge of your hand just above the top of the little finger, lightly on the ledge, before resting your thumb along the thumb ridge.
- Next, curl your fingers around the handle, noting that the back of the thumb ridge does not allow them to wrap too tightly. This will stop you over-gripping, which can make the poles sit too vertically and compromise your wrist angle. Even if you have long fingers, do not let them go past this ridge; just maintain a loose grip.
- The handles should sit loosely in the hand, with the pole angled so the tip is behind you.

STEP 3

To achieve the correct length on the poles:

- Loosen the twist-lock or quick-lock lever so the two parts of the pole can move up and down.
- Start with the pole so it is obviously too high – begin with the handle considerably higher than your elbow when the poles are upright.
- Hold the handle using the step 2 instructions above.
- Stand comfortably upright with feet hip-width apart and toes front facing, with your upper arm by your side and your elbow pulled in to your waist. Place the tip of the pole by the side of your midfoot. Keeping the pole touching the ground, lightly push the handle down until your wrist is level with your elbow. At this point, your forearm will be horizontal and your elbow will be bent at 90 degrees.
- Without lifting the pole from the ground, extend your hand directly forward, away from your body. The pole will now be angled slightly backwards towards your foot, and your arm will be in a similar position to the 'triangle' forward swing position achieved when walking with good posture and awareness.
- If you have set the poles at the best height for you, your wrist will remain straight as you move from 'elbow at your side' to 'elbow straight'. Once you are happy, tighten the poles.

If you feel the pressure between your palm and the handle change as you extend your hand away, the pole is too short. Adjust the pole to be longer and try again.

STEP 4

Warm up (see page 69), but this time practise the movements while holding the poles, rather than placing your hands on your knees for support.

To go to a webpage with free instructions and videos for each of these steps, scan this QR code:

FEELING THE POWER

Now let's explore the power you get from fitness poles.

- Hold the poles in both hands, making sure they are in the right hands and you are gripping the handles correctly.
- Bend your arms at 90 degrees (square position) and push down into the poles. You will feel a little core activation as you do so.
- Next, straighten your arms so your hands are held out as if you want to use both of them to shake hands (triangle position – still holding the poles).
- Now press into the poles. Notice how much greater the core engagement is when your arms are straighter.

Note: The squares and triangles principle is one of the most fundamental ways to get more out of every step. Get it right and you will work the core and improve posture very quickly. The essence of total body walking is to harness larger muscles and engage the core with every step. Bent arms negate this and only work the biceps.

GETTING STARTED WITH FITNESS POLES

With your arms in this straighter position, start to walk forward, ensuring the pole shafts are angled back behind you as you are aiming to get forward propulsion from the poles.

At this point, just get used to walking with the poles, allowing the tips to hit the ground as you swing your arm from the shoulder.

You will feel awkward at first, but just relax and try not to think about the poles, apart from ensuring they are in the correct position. If you feel uncomfortable or out of rhythm, you probably are. Just stop and start again until it feels more natural and relaxed. You should feel as if you are walking with good posture and awareness, but now have longer arms that you can push into the ground (think of the poles as your lower arms and the handles as the elbow joints).

If you feel comfortable, move to total body walking practice exercise 1, below. If you don't, check that you are using opposite arms to legs. This should come naturally, but if you are an overthinker, it may not (if you continue to feel uncomfortable, see page 83 for troubleshooting advice).

TOTAL BODY WALKING PRACTICE EXERCISE 1

Before you begin, follow the sequence above to get started with fitness poles and walk until you feel at ease with them.

- Next, lift the tips off the ground so the poles are still in your hands and angled back, but do not engage with the ground.
- Continue for 10 steps or so and reintroduce the poles. Think about allowing the power of your upper body to transfer into the pole handle via your hand.
- Repeat this process and ask yourself if you can feel a difference:
  o You should feel lighter on your feet and some forward propulsion when the poles engage with the ground.
  o You should also feel slightly faster when using the poles.
  o If you do not, see the troubleshooting advice on page 83 as you may need to recheck your arm position, pole length or how you are using the poles.

If you can feel some power, it's time to build on this.

TOTAL BODY WALKING PRACTICE EXERCISE 2

Now that you have mastered the arm action, it's time to concentrate on your feet and the part they play in boosting your overall fitness.

- Start walking with the poles as described on page 81, keeping your arms straight and your core slightly engaged.

Note: If you are walking with good posture and awareness, your heel touches the ground and you should be rolling through the sole of the foot, finishing with your toes.

- Now keep that action, but consciously push off from your toes as you plant the walking poles into the ground. You should feel an extra push and if your posture is good, an increased lengthening and engagement through the core.
- Practise switching the process of pushing off from your toes on and off a few times.
- Make sure that when you push, you gain forward propulsion, feel your core engage, seem taller and speed up. You should also be smiling. If you aren't, see the troubleshooting advice on page 83.

If you can feel the difference this push off from the toes has to the whole-body engagement, you are ready for the total body walking practice exercise 3, but I would also advise that you go for a walk trying to maintain this action. You will feel it in the core and arms and will begin to feel breathless too.

TOTAL BODY WALKING PRACTICE EXERCISE 3

Now it is time to increase the intensity, at least for short bursts, until you can maintain it for every step. This action is where the calorie-burning intensity that total body pole walking can give you is coming into play. It is about effort and will need practice before you can maintain it.

- Concentrate on the push through the pole handle, which should happen at the same time as the feet roll through for the push-off.
- Rather than pushing *harder* through the handle, think about pushing *longer*, allowing the pole tip to stay in contact with the ground longer as you roll through the foot, engage the core and

step forward with the other leg. It is easy to fall into simply tapping poles into the ground and not *using* them.

- Practise pushing into the handle and off the toes before relaxing and walking with less effort, but good form. Repeat several times and you will be getting an interval workout as well as mastering total body walking.

TIP

A good way to think about this action when practising is to imagine the poles are pushing a doorbell or buzzer. A short sharp buzz or a longer buzzzzzzzz!

TOTAL BODY WALKING PRACTICE EXERCISE 4

Using your poles as per the three previous exercises, try moving up through the paces outlined on page 53, from postural (exertion rate: 3/10) to purposeful (5/10) and then building up with the longer push described above to reach performance pace (9/10). You are now total body walking.

TROUBLESHOOTING ADVICE

The following are common mistakes that can be made when walking with poles to prevent total body walking from occurring: lack of coordination, using a square-arm action or using poles that are too long or too short. Here's how to counteract them.

LACK OF COORDINATION

Coordination is key to a natural rhythmic action that gives propulsion. It also helps to keep you balanced and encourages healthy rotation of the spine. However, as soon as we start to think about which arm should go forward with each foot we tend to become stiff and move strangely. For that reason, when teaching I tend to not mention coordination.

The best way to tackle poor coordination is to simply walk and forget any arm movement. Clear your mind and concentrate only on your steps. Then become aware of your arms. Note that they swing gently in time with the opposite leg (when you are not thinking about them or holding poles).

Now replicate this sequence, but hold the poles gently and allow them to drag behind you. Once again, clear your mind and, when you become aware of your arms, imagine the poles are not there. Think about simply walking as described, gently allowing your arms to swing to handshake height with the poles following behind. If at any point this becomes stiff or uncoordinated, stop and start again.

Once you have mastered this, try to follow the planting and pushing actions outlined in total body walking practice exercise 3 (see page 82). If you notice your arms and legs have lost coordination at any time, restart this whole sequence again.

The common reason for loss of coordination is that people immediately alter their leg speed once their arms come into play, so another good exercise is to count steps to a beat, making sure the rhythm does not change once you introduce an arm-swing movement.

SQUARE-ARM ACTION WITH A BENT ELBOW

This common fault often occurs simply because our instant reaction to poles is to grip them tightly and use them with a bent arm, as you might use a walking stick. Typically, it will take practice to maintain the swing from the shoulder (a triangle action – see page 79). For some people, this may be too difficult to start with, because they do not have the fitness levels to use so many major muscles in unison.

The long arm swing and stride might literally be a step too far, so if you feel you are bending your arms because it's easier to breathe comfortably, take things slowly and try to maintain a good arm swing, but only for short practice exercises. Build up your fitness walking without poles rather than falling into using poles with a bent arm action.

POLES ARE TOO LONG

If your poles are too long, it will affect the pole plant angle, which in turn will affect propulsion and tip engagement with the floor. It also affects the grip and wrist angle due to the pole angle (as detailed above).

There are a few signs to look out for:

• If you are struggling with getting a clear pole plant (especially if the pole feels like it is slipping), can't get the grip right or your wrists feel uncomfortable, check your pole setting.

- If you have rubber ferrules or 'paws' on the bottom of your fitness poles, they will wear out on one edge if the poles are too long, so check for uneven wear towards the front of the paws.
- Try adjusting the poles by 1cm (½in) at a time until the action and pole plant feel more natural and comfortable.

POLES ARE TOO SHORT

When your poles are too short it becomes difficult to gain propulsion and you will find that you dip forwards from your shoulders as you plant the poles. Alternatively, you will not achieve a good arm swing, because the pole lifts too far off the ground when your hand reaches handshake height and you feel rushed into planting it. The poles will generally be too far forwards and cause the dipping action mentioned above, and you may feel you tend to 'misplant'. This will cause wear towards the back of a rubber paw. As with poles that are too long, try adjusting your poles by 1cm (½in) at a time and evaluate the change. You will notice a huge difference when you get the height right.

Element 2: Strength and tone exercises

As I outlined in Chapter 4 (see page 60), there are four basic moves which are the foundation of strength training and do not require any kit. Below I explain how to do each one safely. Let's start with the ultimate lower-body exercises – squats and lunges.

1. Squats

If I only did one strength exercise it would be this one. It is so beneficial because it uses all the major upper-body skeletal muscles, providing strength and stability through to the core and spine. It's also a good calorie-burner and helps to keep you supple. Finally, it can be done pretty much anywhere, so is great as your staple walking strengthener. Simply stop walking and perform a few squats once you are nice and warm and in an appropriate spot. You can also play around with sets of steps and squats to keep it fun, for example 20 steps and 2 squats for a section of your walk. There are more ideas to follow.

Note: If you feel any discomfort in your lower back while squatting, you may prefer to start with lunges as your main leg strengthener.

HOW TO SQUAT

The aim of a squat is to bend the knees, lowering your bodyweight, and then stand back up slowly, working the muscles in different ways on the up and down movements. The key is to perform them in a controlled manner and not to overdo it.

- Good form is to stand with your feet hip-distance apart and facing forward.
- Keep your knees in line with each other as you lower your weight down towards your heels.
- Keep a good strong spine and note that your shoulders will come forward slightly as you push your bottom back.
- Make sure your feet are still anchored on the ground and your knees do not go over your toes.
- Stand up, taking the same time as you took to drop down, as every movement is working one set of muscles.

How deep you go on a squat is mainly based on your personal hip, knee and ankle mobility, so aim for as low as you can manage without taking your heels off the ground or allowing your bottom to drop lower than the knees – if that's not very low, don't worry, just keep practising. A good 90-degree angle at the knee with thighs parallel to the ground is spot on, if you can get there.

HOW MANY SQUATS?

If you are a beginner, aim to do 10 repetitions if you can (if you can't, then build up to 10). Rest and then attempt some more (ideally the same number of repetitions as you managed in the last set).

A good amount to keep your muscles in great condition is three sets of 10 or 12 repetitions. Once that becomes easy, you can look at the advanced exercises on page 103 to keep challenging yourself.

'Life has its ups and downs – we call them squats!'

2. Lunges

Lunges are fantastic, because they work both sides of the body in a different way, without putting too much strain on the back. Using the major muscles in the front and back of the legs and your derrière, they are good calorie-burners and are great for balance and coordination too.

Like squats, lunges are perfect for inserting into a walk and you can work up to bursts of forward or reverse step lunges. The best way to master them is to learn the static movement at home first. Then master how to incorporate a forward or backward step and you will soon be lunge-walking and adding twists.

HOW TO LUNGE

There are three types of lunges: static lunges, which are great for mastering stability in the movement, and forward and reverse step lunges that you can incorporate on the go in your daily walks. This variety will target your body in different ways.

STATIC LUNGES

- Stand with your feet hip-width apart – hands clasped together at chest height – and step forward with one leg.
- Take the other leg back with a slightly longer step so you are in a split stance.
- You are now in the best position to check your lunge positioning – this is crucial when you begin to step into them with walking lunges.
- Keep the core strong with good posture and relaxed shoulders.
- Lower your body so both knees are at a 90-degree angle – you will need to go on to the toes of the rear leg.
- Take care not to let the lead knee go out of line with the ankle.
- Hold this position briefly before slowly pulling back up to the split stance.
- Repeat with the same lead leg before switching the stance, so the legs have both been challenged equally in lead and rear positions.

Once you have mastered the leg positions at the lower point in the movement above and are confident with your stability, you can try stepping straight into the lunges.

Note: If stationary or step lunges cause discomfort to your knees, check out the reverse step lunge below.

FORWARD STEP LUNGE

- Stand with your feet hip-width apart – hands clasped together at chest height – and take a step forward with one leg, dropping into the lunge position outlined in the static lunge above.
- Come up out of the lunge by stepping back to the start position with the other leg each time.
- Repeat with the same leg before changing to alternate legs. This will challenge your coordination.

REVERSE STEP LUNGE

This is a similar move to the forward step lunge, but this time you take a step backwards. The results are similar in that the end movement is the same, but this type of lunge is easier on the lead knee because when we step forward we are also putting a braking force through that lead knee. When we do the reverse lunge, the lead knee is stationary, so it experiences less force.

Note: If you feel unstable when lunging, you may want to start off with squats (see page 85) as your main leg strengthener.

HOW MANY LUNGES?

Aim to perform 10 repetitions and try to repeat that two or three times so you build up to three sets of 10 or 12.

3. Press-ups

Now it's time to move on to simple ways to work the upper body. Most of us know what a press-up (or push-up) is, but as they usually involve getting on to the ground, these adapted versions are suitable for performing outdoors, when out walking in all weathers. As well as an incline press-up there are alternative standing versions with a wide or narrow grip, which are perfect for outdoors as it is often easier to find something to press against that is at least chest height – trees are perfect. This also involves no bending at the start.

Press-ups are beneficial because they use all the major upper-body skeletal muscles, providing strength and stability through the chest, shoulders, back of the arms and upper back. Because they involve so many muscles, they also have a calorie-burning effect. These versions can be done pretty much anywhere and are slightly easier than traditional press-ups.

HOW TO DO INCLINE PRESS-UPS

By incline I simply mean that rather than having your body flat on the ground and pushing it up, you seek out a bench, log or other fixture in a park or the great outdoors. You need something that is stable and ideally between knee and waist height. The lower your platform is, the harder the press-ups will be as you are asking your arms to lift the weight of your upper body further.

- Select a bench, wall, rail, fence or tree stump and place your hands on it – palms down and fingers facing forward, about one and a half shoulder widths apart.
- Keep your arms straight, holding your bodyweight. Bend your knees slightly, with your feet as far from the platform you are using as is comfortable.
- Your elbows are going to come out to the sides as you take your arms down to a 90-degree angle. Try to keep your upper arms in line with the bench or rail.
- Bring your chest as low as you comfortably can, keeping your back nice and straight. Look slightly ahead, rather than down, to keep your neck strong.
- Now push the floor away from you until you fully extend your arms.
- If you feel comfortable, repeat this action with straighter legs. This increases the effectiveness of the press-up, as you have what is termed a 'longer lever'.
- Repeat as many press-ups as you can with your knees in the best position for you.

HOW TO DO STANDING OR UPRIGHT PRESS-UPS (WIDE GRIP)

- Find a tree or upright object that can bear being pushed against and lean into it.

- Make sure you take your feet far enough away to cause you to lean into the tree/object with bent arms. Ensure your feet are flat on the ground and stable.
- Place your hands on the tree/object using a nice wide hand grip, similar to the previous incline press-up, but slightly wider, about two shoulder-widths apart if you have the room on your object.
- Take your elbows out to a 90-degree angle as you take your chest down towards the tree/object.
- Now push the tree/object away from you until you fully extend your arms.
- As you do the exercise, try to move your body as one unit. Keep your head up so that your ears are above your shoulders.

TIP

I like to do press-ups against trees because you can connect with them at the same time.

HOW MANY PRESS-UPS?

Aim to perform 10 repetitions. Try to repeat that two or three times, so you build up to three sets of 10 or 12.

4. Triceps dips

The ultimate bodyweight arm exercise, dips can be challenging, but are effective. They mainly target the back of the arms, but are a good core activator too.

HOW TO DO TRICEPS DIPS

- Select a platform such as a bench, low wall, log or other fixture in a park – ideally one you can sit on at the start and when at rest between sets. Make sure there is room for your upper body to drop down towards the floor in front of it.
- Sit on the platform and place your hands on to the edge, with either knees bent and feet flat on the ground or legs straight with your weight resting on the heels (the latter makes the exercise harder).

- Move forward to take your weight on to straight arms. Your fingers should be facing your buttocks. Stay close to the platform to protect your wrists.
- Lower your buttocks and legs towards the ground as one unit, making sure your elbows are pointing straight back behind you at 90 degrees, not out to the sides.
- Make sure your core is engaged and keep your shoulders close to your ears. Stop if you experience any shoulder discomfort.
- Come back up slowly.
- Repeat before sitting back down and taking the weight off your arms.

HOW MANY TRICEPS DIPS?

Aim to perform 10 repetitions and try to repeat that two or three times, so you build up to three sets of 10 or 12.

TIP

A simple way to add resistance training to a walk is to make use of the outdoor gyms found in many parks, which are typically free.

For a full range of more advanced strength workouts and variations based on these four basic moves, see the advanced exercises on page 108.

Element 3: Balance, flexibility and range of movement exercises

These static balance exercises are ideal for working on the third element of fitness. Start indoors and close to something to hold on to at first, but build a habit that works for you. Some people advocate doing balance exercises while brushing their teeth or waiting for the kettle to boil, for instance. I think including a balance sequence in a walk (especially where other elements are included) is the fastest, most effective way to make sure you do not skip them. Walk to a favourite spot and run through the balance sequence while fixing your eyes on something that is lovely *but* still! See the standing yoga poses (page 31) for other great flexibility and balance exercises.

(page 31)

Safety tips for balance exercises

- -

Wear smooth-soled shoes and start slowly. If you have poor balance initially, keep your weight over your ankles. Be aware of dizziness and stop immediately if you feel uncomfortable, especially if you are on medication for hypertension or similar. If you have experienced vertigo or labyrinthitis or have any medical condition that affects balance, take extra care and work within your abilities with a stable object to hand at all times to hold on to if needed.

Static balance practice exercise for indoors or outside

This exercise can be done both indoors and outdoors. It is a simple way to get the leg muscles used to your bodyweight shifting as you balance. One way to remember to do it is to use it to pop your socks or shoes on.

- Stand beside a worktop, chair or bench. Keep your non-dominant hand ready to grab this surface to steady yourself if you wobble.
- Start by just asking one leg to take your weight as you lift the other one, bending your knee at 90 degrees in front of you. Your arms should be by your sides but not moving. If you need to, though, take them outwards at shoulder height.
- Take a minute to check in with the leg that you are standing on. Feel how your ankle and lower leg muscles adjust to this position.
- If you feel you can challenge the leg more – raise your arms up or out to change your centre of gravity slightly.
- Repeat, lifting the other leg.
- To add difficulty, stand on one leg as above, but bend down and pretend to put a sock on the lifted foot.

Static balance sequence 1

This is a more advanced sequence, which is best performed outdoors where possible as you need more space than for the exercise above. The great outdoors also provides slopes, cambers, slippery and soft surfaces to contend with, making balance more challenging. Initially, having something to grab if needed is advised. Using fitness poles is great as you can choose to use one or two and even lift them off the ground, but be ready to use them if needed.

- Keep your non-dominant hand ready to grab the rail, poles or bench you are using to steady yourself if you wobble.
- Start by just asking the leg to take the weight, then lift this leg, bending the knee at 90 degrees. Your arms should be by your sides but not moving, but if you need to, take them outwards at shoulder height.
- Take a minute to check in with the leg that you are standing on. Feel how your ankle and lower leg muscles adjust to this position.
- Turn your head slowly to each side. Try looking upwards and see how that adds a small challenge to the process.
- Repeat, lifting the other leg.
- To add difficulty, try closing your eyes as you hold the balance on one leg.

Static balance sequence 2

Follow the instructions above to stand on one leg. If you feel you can, challenge the leg more by raising your arms up or out to change your centre of gravity slightly. Then take your lifted leg through a series of movements that change your centre of gravity, while keeping your arms out to the sides:

- Straighten your lifted leg and point your toes in front of you (keeping them off the ground, if you can).
- Slowly take your straight leg out to the side. If it feels more comfortable, you can keep your knee bent.
- Take your lifted leg behind you and point it backwards. Lean slightly forwards, if you can.
- Bring the lifted leg back to the raised starting position before placing it back down.
- Repeat, lifting the other leg.

Static balance sequence 3

In this version we change the body position more, which sends even more messages to the anchor leg.

- Follow the leg sequence above. This time, when you take your leg behind you try to lean as far forward as you can, taking your leg up behind you into an 'arabesque' pose with your arms out to the sides.
- Try raising your arms or adjusting their position.
- Gently come back up to standing and pull the lifted leg through to the front before placing it down.
- Repeat, lifting the other leg.
- To add difficulty, place something soft on the ground between your legs, which you have to step over as you change legs.

For a range of moving balance exercises, see the fitness walking sequences that follow. Most of these will challenge balance in some way, but you can also experiment with pausing on a walk and standing on one leg – maybe add a few boxing punches, punching the arms slightly across the body and alternating between the left and right. You could also progress from standing to stepping, pausing and punching. Another great idea is to hover over a step as you climb a flight of them or step up a kerb with a pause before you transfer your weight.

TIP

Balance pods or pads are a great way to add a challenge to balance exercises as they provide an unstable surface.

Fitness walking sequences

These are simple exercise sequences that can incorporate all three elements of fitness that your body needs: cardiovascular; strength and tone; and balance, flexibility and range of movement. The sequences gradually increase in difficulty and intensity to keep you challenged.

They save you having to think about what to do and they can be done at any time, mid-walk or on a specific workout walk.

Use the fitness walking sequences as a fun way to build strength, balance and range of movement into your walking. Pick and choose the sequences to add variety and to challenge your mind and body, and work your way as far through them as you can. Don't worry if you are not able to complete (or remember) all the phases initially – you will build up your strength, range of movement and balance quickly if you persist and the sequence moves will become second nature. If you are also adding other fitness exercises, try to add sequences to at least one walk a week. If time is short, master the sequences that are most relevant for your goals and try to add them to four walks a week. Simply repeating them twice and adding the progressions will be a great starting point and will soon make a difference. Most of the sequences work well with fitness poles, too, which is a great way to make a short walk very effective.

The tightrope sequence – for balance and leg strength

If you have a painted line available (perhaps along the side of a sports pitch or quiet road), you can use this to create a moving balance exercise.

1 Walk normally with your usual stride length, but place one foot directly in front of the other on the line ahead. Continue for a few steps.
2 Add some difficulty by reducing your step length, placing the heel of your foot directly against the toes of the foot already on the line and repeating. You may need to place your hands out to the sides.
3 Add more difficulty by returning your stride to normal, but dipping into a semi-squat position as you continue to walk on the line.
4 If you can, continue with the walking squat, but as you take each leg forward, allow it to hover with your knee bent before placing it down and performing the squat. This further challenges your balance.
5 The final movement will change your body position, so make sure you are ready for it! As you come up out of the squat, lift your back leg behind you as you tilt your body forward (from the hip not the back). Pull the leg through to the bent knee hover described above before placing it on the line. Repeat with the other leg.

The crab walk sequence – for strength, coordination and impact

This sequence strengthens the legs and targets muscles not used fully when moving forward. It also boosts coordination and range of movement and can strengthen bones too.

1 Turn to face the right-hand side of the path. Take a side or crab lunge step with your left leg, nice and wide. Keep your knees and feet at a 10 and 2 o'clock angle so they stay aligned. Keep your glutes back, and your back straight and low. Take around 10 steps, then turn to the left-hand side and repeat the side lunges with your right leg.

2 Bring in some coordination. After one crab lunge with your left leg, rotate so you're leading with your right leg, with your left leg facing the opposite direction. Continue, rotating with every lunge to lead with alternate legs.

3 Bring in some impact. Rather than taking a slow step, bounce to one side, taking two steps with less of a squat. Add a little swing to your arms, keeping them out to the side as you gallop from one side to the other.

The puppet master sequence – for balance and coordination

This fitness walking sequence is purely designed to challenge balance and coordination when walking. It's a fun one to do, but it does work better in a group where you don't know what you will be asked to do next. If you are with somebody else, take it in turns to be the 'puppet master' – this adds to the challenge element of the sequence.

1 Start by walking normally, then imagine you have strings attached to your major joints and these are controlled by a puppet master.

2 Lift each leg to a square 90-degree position as you step forward with it – pausing slightly with the leg in the air and taking weight on to the other leg before placing it back down.

3 Bring in the arms. Keep them straight with your hands on your thighs to start, then, if you can, lift them out in front of you at

shoulder height with each step. Check you are working opposite arms and legs.

4 Challenge that by pausing and lifting the arm and leg on the *same* side.

5 Switch back and forth from opposites to the same side (as if the puppet master is practising).

6 Repeat the process, taking the arms straight up above the head with the upper arms close to the ears.

7 If you feel you can, try to bounce slightly from leg to leg in a more dynamic way for a few paces as you lift those arms high.

8 Bring the walk back down to the basic movements when you are ready.

The subway sequence – for strength, balance and coordination

This sequence helps you to adapt your centre of gravity, and maintain good posture as you drop your weight down and walk on your toes.

1 Walk forward, starting in an upright position.

2 Begin to lower your body, keeping your back straight as you gradually drop into a walking lunge position (imagining you are going down into a subway).

3 Continue walking in this lower position.

4 Gradually begin to straighten up with each step until you go past the start position. Now begin walking on tiptoes.

5 Drop back down gradually into the starting position and repeat.

The step, squat, lunge and jump shuffle sequence – for strength, coordination and impact

This is a multi-faceted sequence which is designed to target muscles in different ways. The lunge steps and shuffle backs could even be used on their own for a short but effective addition to a walk.

1 Take two big lunge steps forward, keeping your knee over your ankle.

2 Shuffle back quickly using fast steps.

3 Take two more big steps forward and add at least three squats before shuffling back again.

4 This time take a springing jump forward, powered by taking your arms back and bringing them forward as you spring. Land with your weight on your heels before doing at least three squats. Shuffle back as before.

The ski jump sequence – for impact, bone strength and CV

This ski jump sequence is all about impact – it's a great way to up the cardiovascular effect of a walk, too.

1 Stand with your feet hip-distance apart. Go into a squat position by swinging your arms back and bending your knees.

2 As you drive your arms forward, *jump* with both feet. Make sure that you land with bent knees and your weight on your heels.

The backwards walking sequence – for balance and coordination

Challenge your brain and muscles more with this simple exercise that can also include bursts of speed to increase the CV effects.

1 Make sure you have a clear path behind you. Begin walking backwards, pushing off from your toes and feeling your leg muscles working differently.

2 Take 10 steps backwards before rotating to take 10 steps forwards. Keep repeating the switch, taking care to push off from your toes on the backward phase and to start with your heel on the forwards phase.

3 Practise step 1 on an incline with a jog or brisk walk forwards to the starting point.

4 Practise step 2 by switching between backwards and forwards walking, but on an incline. Return to the starting point. If the incline is not too steep you can alternate or simply walk briskly back.

The speed skater sequence – for range of movement, impact, strength and balance

This sequence is for mastering how to adapt strides, balance and steps for uneven ground.

1 Take a big step forward on the diagonal, away from the centre line. Make sure your weight goes into your heel and your lead knee stays bent, above the ankle.
2 Tilt your body forward slightly and swing your arms from side to side like a skater, tapping the back leg behind you before stepping it forward to repeat.
3 Continue with the wide step and arm swings, but this time don't tap the back leg on the ground. Hover with it bent before stepping through to repeat. If you can, add a small impact as you land on each leg.
4 Repeat the step and arm action, but this time extend the rear leg behind you and straighten it, leaning forward as you pause to balance for a second before pulling it through to take the next step. You can choose whether to use impact or a smooth step.

The forward-travelling lunge sequence – for strength, balance, range of movement and coordination

A perfect all-rounder, this sequence brings the upper body into play and is great for building up leg and core strength for walking on uneven ground.

1 Perform forward lunge steps (see page 88), taking your knees to a 90-degree bend, if possible. Alternate the legs to travel forward as you do so, keeping your hands on your hips.
2 To increase the challenge, bring your arms into play. Bring them up so the fingers of both hands meet in front of the chest with elbows out to the sides, nice and high. Continue lunge-stepping in this position.
3 This time take your arms up over your head, interlocking your fingers and keeping your arms straight. This changes your bodyweight and

challenges your range of movement in your upper body, as well as your balance. Continue lunge-stepping in this position.

4 To challenge your coordination, simply alternate between the two arm positions with every other step.

The backward lunge sequence – for leg strength and balance

Challenge your coordination and ability to adjust to a change in your centre of gravity as you strengthen your legs.

1 Take a big step back with one leg – push your toes into the ground and keep your heel raised. Try to get both knees as close to a 90-degree angle as you can and keep your posture up. Next, take your other leg back and alternate for 10 steps.

2 Repeat the same action, but work one leg at a time, performing about 10 steps on one side before swapping over.

3 This takes some coordination. Take your large lunge back as far as you can and travel backwards with each lunge. Keep your chest up nice and high, and take your bodyweight down until your knees are at a 90-degree angle. Make sure the path behind you is clear.

4 To increase the challenge, bring your arms into play. Start with them close to your chest and your elbows pointing downwards. As you take the lunge step, take them out straight in front of you at chest height and return as you complete each lunge. Be careful as this challenges your balance. You could also try taking your elbows out to the sides and pushing forward with your hands, keeping your elbows high (like a chest press action with each lunge).

The bum kicks sequence – for balance and range of movement

This exercise works the hamstrings, and the knees experience a fuller range of movement.

1 Walk forward with the backs of your hands on your lower buttocks.

2 Kick your back leg up behind you and try to get your foot as close to your hand as possible. Continue with alternate legs as you walk.

3 Take this further by adding bounces or hops for impact.

The upright chest press-up sequence – for strength

The next couple of sequences require something to sit on or push against as they bring the upper body into play. Walking and running are great ways to exercise outdoors, but upper body strength can be neglected. Getting into the habit of adding these will ensure you do not lose tone and upper-body strength. It will also ensure you have the arm strength to break a fall. (Please note, this exercise has already been described on page 89.)

1. Stand facing a tree or wall. Place a nice wide hand grip on to it, taking your elbows out to a 90-degree angle as you take your chest down towards the surface.
2. Keep pressing and straightening your arms, making sure as you do the exercise that you try to move your body as one unit. Keep your head up with your ears above your shoulders.
3. Repeat but with a narrower grip, so your hands are only shoulder-width apart and your elbows come towards your waist.
4. Alternate between the wide and narrow grips for a greater workout of the chest area. Remember, your torso needs to stay nice and straight.

For a horizontal chest press-up sequence, follow the steps above using a log or a bench (see page 88).

The triceps bench sequence

If you work the biceps via the press-ups above, it's always best to do something to target the opposing muscles in the upper arm for even tone and to avoid imbalance. This exercise tones the backs of the arms, which are often a problem area.

1. Follow the directions for a triceps dips (see page 91), using a bench or log.
2. Start with your legs bent to make this movement easier to perform.
3. Straighten both legs, resting your weight on your heels to add a degree of difficulty.
4. This time, straighten one leg at a time with each press. This adds some core engagement as you work to avoid your body twisting.

Reading through these exercises and trying to remember them all at once is a tall order, but I promise that if you practise them one at a time, they soon become second nature. Not only will you be able to perform them more easily, but you'll be able to do more each time, and you will even be able to start making up your own sequences. You will also notice that you feel stronger, move better and enjoy the variety. Once you get to that point, it's time to challenge yourself further and add some more ways to ensure you keep progressing. That's what we're going to tackle next.

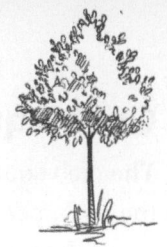

6

WALK THIS WAY...
To take it further with maximum fitness sequences

If you have enjoyed incorporating basic exercises into your walks as outlined in the previous chapter, here are some more advanced versions to add variety, avoid boredom and keep you progressing. They will also help you to create your own fitness walking sequences.

In this chapter we build strength by learning variations on the squat and lunge. We then look at how to add to the usual press-ups to work different muscles, and cover advanced upper-body exercises to push our muscles even harder. Finally, we discover how to enhance our use of walking poles when out and about. Any kit we use is fully portable and once you are confident enough to introduce these additions, you can truly create your own personal walking gym!

The following challenge your body more, for example by incorporating changes in direction. I call them total body walking exercises.

Squat variations

Master these squat variations to target your muscles in different ways and gain an understanding of how you can build simple sequences into your walking workouts.

Crab squat

The crab squat is a great travelling squat as you can turn to the side of the path, perform a set and then keep shuffling forwards. These squats target the buttocks and upper thighs.

- Turn to the side. Take a step out laterally from that side in the direction you were walking, squatting normally with both legs as you do so.
- Bring both legs together and stand back up, before taking another crab squat step to the same side. Repeat.
- Turn to face the opposite direction so the other leg is now stepping you forward along the path ahead and repeat on the other side.

Stay-low crab shuffle

This is similar to the crab squat above, but the stay-low crab shuffle is more about the side movement than the squat. It is great for a walking workout as you keep going forward.

- Take a squat position and, once dropped down, hold.
- Take small side steps while in this position, before standing up.
- Turn to face the opposite direction and do the same with the other leg leading.

Sumo squat

With two slight changes to the basic squat, the targeted muscles change. Use them to spice up your squats or add to a sequence.

- Simply widen the starting squat stance so your legs are wider than your hips.
- Turn your toes out, so you are squatting like a sumo wrestler about to fight.
- Come back up slowly as before and repeat.

Single-leg squat

Only attempt these once you know you can perform a squat without knee pain. If you are not sure about your ability to balance, perform it beside something you can grab to stabilise yourself (park benches are great for this).

- Lift one leg off the ground slightly in front of you and perform the squats with the other leg, paying attention to posture and balance.
- You could add further variation by taking the lifted leg to the side or behind you (see the balance sequences on page 91). Do as many as you feel comfortable with and always repeat with the other leg.

Curtsy squat

If you can do the sumo and single-leg squats, try the curtsy – an elegant move perfected by those who meet royalty. It also mirrors what we tend to do when we bend to pick something up from the ground and is in essence half squat, half lunge.

- Bend both knees. As you lower your body, take one leg diagonally behind you so it crosses the body.
- Using your toes, position this leg so the knee is just off the ground.
- Maintain good posture and a strong core throughout as you try to keep the thigh of the squatting leg parallel to the ground.
- Repeat with the other leg.

Skater squat

This squat is tougher on the legs, and requires more balance and coordination.

- Start in the lower part of the squat position and take one leg out behind you but to one side, as if you are skating along.
- Hold the outstretched leg there as you straighten up.
- Take your arms out wide and hold this three-pointed star pose before squatting back down.
- Repeat if you can and remember to do the same on the other leg.

TIP

If time is short, the squat is a perfect base to combine upper- and lower-body strength exercises. See the upper-body exercises on page 109.

Squat variations with resistance

The following incorporate more resistance, usually via some kind of fitness equipment rather than just bodyweight.

SQUAT WITH BAND

The easiest, most convenient way to add resistance to a squat on the move is via resistance bands. If only working on the legs, use a fabric band just above the knees. Perform the squat as usual, but push out against the band as you do so to work the outside of the thighs. Holding the bands in the hands can turn the squat into a combination exercise too.

SQUAT WITH WEIGHT

Adding weight to the squat means you are asking the leg muscles to work against more resistance. You can make this simple by just holding something of a manageable size and weight at waist height as you perform the squat, or slightly change position, as outlined in the next two moves.

SUITCASE SQUAT

This time, hold a weight (I use sand-filled neoprene weights, but small dumbbells or weighted balls would work too – it depends on what you find easiest to pop in your pack if you want to carry them with you) in each hand, keeping your arms at the side of your body and starting with your hands around your knees. Perform your squat – this takes your arms towards the ground and back to the starting point. Imagine you are lifting two suitcases from the ground with straight arms.

Lunge variations

These lunge variations include changes in direction and leg positioning. Lunges are the ultimate sequence exercise, so once you master them take a look at the sequences on page 99 to turn them into dynamic super-moves.

Lunge with a twist

Simply twist your torso to one side as you perform any of the lunge variations. Always twist to the side of the lead leg and back before returning to the start position. Remember to switch the twist as you switch the lead leg. To add to the effectiveness, hold your arms straight out in front of you.

Elevated leg lunge (front)

This lunge can be done on steps or low benches. Elevating the lead leg can make it easier on the knees, so this is great for beginners.

- Put the whole of your *front* foot on to a step, making sure you have full support.
- Perform the lunge until your thigh on your lead leg is parallel to the floor.
- Repeat with the other leg.

Elevated leg lunge (rear)

This one is tougher and works the front of the elevated leg as well as the lunging leg.

- Place the back foot on to the bench.
- Perform the lunge, keeping the back leg in that position.
- Repeat with the other leg.

Lunge variations with resistance

These lunges use alternative resistance from equipment, not just your bodyweight.

LUNGES WITH WEIGHT

Holding something heavy across your front will add intensity to the legs during any of the above lunges. Always maintain good lunge form.

SUITCASE LUNGE

For this lunge, hold a weight in each hand and hang your arms down beside your body. Perform any of the lunge variations, keeping your arms straight as you lower the weights towards the floor, as if you were placing two suitcases down. As you straighten or step back up, you will be lifting the 'suitcases' off the ground, adding to the resistance.

BANDED LUNGES

Using a wider fabric lunge band placed just above the knees, take a step back into a lunge, pulling against the band. You can perform a few on each leg in turn or alternate.

Press-up variations

These press-up variations challenge the muscles in different ways.

Narrow grip incline press-up

This version increases the intensity and works the arms differently. It's a great strengthener for those who aim to use fitness poles in their total body walking.

- Repeat the exercise for incline press-ups (see page 89). This time, start by placing your hands at shoulder-width.
- As you lower your body towards the platform, you need to keep your arms to the sides this time, bringing your elbows to your waist as you do the 90-degree bend.
- Once again you can choose a short lever with a knee bend or, if you can, straighten the legs to increase intensity.

Narrow grip standing or upright press-up

As with the incline press, you can repeat the standing or upright press (see page 89) with a narrower hand placement and arm angle. Your hands should be only shoulder-width apart and your elbows should come towards your waist. Alternating between grips gives a two-in-one workout effect.

Single arm press-up

A great way to add intensity to a press-up in any format is to do it on one arm only. As you are putting much more bodyweight or resistance into one limb, it is vital that you have mastered good form when performing press-ups to avoid straining the muscles involved.

Advanced upper-body exercises using resistance

Working the smaller upper-body muscles against resistance rather than bodyweight on the go is best done with resistance bands. You can read more about them on page 135.

Triceps band exercise

Select a loop band that you can stretch comfortably for this exercise.

- Stand with your feet shoulder-width apart.
- Place the loop over one wrist and place that hand on the opposite shoulder with your arm crossing your chest.
- Hold the other end of the band with the opposite hand. Keeping the band in place at the shoulder, pull it backwards until the arm on the working side is straight at the elbow. Keep your wrist firm.
- Repeat on this side about 10 times, before repeating on the other side.

Bicep curl band exercise

To perform a standing bicep curl, which works the front of the arm, you will need a longer band. If you only have loop bands, try sitting on a bench and putting the loops under your feet as this will work in the same way. Use either a section of band that is cut to length or a band with handles on, which will make the grip and hand position more comfortable.

- Stand with your feet shoulder-width apart and place a band under them. Make sure you have an equal amount of excess band on either side.
- Pick up the band ends or handles and start on one side, with your hand beside your thigh.
- Pull the band upwards, ensuring your upper arm remains at the side and your elbow does not move forwards or outwards.
- Pull the band up until your hand is close to your shoulders. Return to the start position in a controlled manner.
- Repeat about 10 times on one side before changing to the other arm and repeating.

Shoulder band exercise

For this exercise, select a loop band that you can stretch comfortably.

- Stand with your feet shoulder-width apart.
- Anchor the band with one hand close to your torso, just below your waist, keeping that arm close to your body.
- Take the other hand and grip the loop of the band.
- Pull the band until it tightens, taking your arm up to shoulder height and outwards to work the shoulder.
- Do not let the band take over. Use controlled movements to pull and lower your hand back to the starting point.
- Repeat about 10 times on this side before changing to the other arm and repeating.

Lateral pull down with looped band

For this exercise, select a loop band that you can stretch comfortably. It is important to keep the band close to the front of your body as this puts less pressure on your shoulders.

- Stand with your feet shoulder-width apart.
- Hold the band in both hands, gripping the looped ends.
- Raise the band above your head.
- Widen the band as you pull it down to chest height, using controlled movements.

TIP

Turn these upper-body exercises into combination moves by adding squats or lunges.

Advanced exercises with fitness poles

Before attempting these more advanced moves, make sure you have used the poles comfortably and confidently for walking, and check your grip and wrist angles are correct.

Using both fitness poles together

To increase the upper-body workout when using fitness poles, plant them both on the ground together.

- Concentrate on the double-powered push, making sure your grip is correct and the wrist angle is not compromised. As you push into both handles, extend your core and roll through your lead foot.
- You may find that it's easier to perform the push only on this leg stride, before switching to the other leg as the lead.
- Alternatively, you can push and take two steps before pushing again.

Bounding or skipping with fitness poles

To add explosive and CV elements plus some impact, you can add a bounding action to your step or skip when using poles.

The advanced exercises in this chapter will help you challenge yourself to achieve higher levels of fitness. Of course, I appreciate that not everyone will want try them all – perhaps they seem daunting and not quite what you thought walking would be about – but even so I encourage you to give them a go. Pick a single exercise, spend some time mastering it and then see where that takes you. You might be surprised!

7

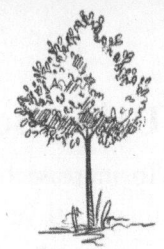

WALK THIS WAY...

To refresh, recoup and recover

There are so many health conditions that leave people feeling exercise is impossible for them, but in over 40 years I have found few conditions that cannot be improved by a well-thought-out walking programme. I don't have space here to go through every condition, but I touch on those where walking can make a difference and point to the most relevant elements of fitness (see Chapter 4) or daily inspirations (see Chapter 10) that can support recovery. Most national organisations and charities also give guidance about suitable exercise for the specific condition they represent.

What follows are some real-life stories of how walking, particularly using fitness poles, has helped people. I also trust that reading the case studies will give hope to those suffering from similar conditions and illustrate the positive effect walking can have on health and well-being.

Note: It is important that if you have a specific condition, you consult your doctor and, where possible, use a qualified exercise referral practitioner before embarking on an exercise regime. If you ask about social prescribing, your doctor might be able to signpost you to a supportive group with walking sessions. Remember to listen to your body and understand what makes it feel better and what may aggravate your condition.

Diabetes

Exercise is one of the most important factors in the management of diabetes and – along with medication and lifestyle advice – can make a huge difference. Walking is one of the most beneficial ways to become more active and has specific properties that make it ideal for both type 1 and type 2 diabetics, as well as those identified as prediabetic – walking is one of the best ways to reduce the risk of developing diabetes too.

If you have diabetes the key element of fitness to include in your walks is CV exercise, but as strength training also helps to reduce body fat and improve metabolism, try to include that in your walks, too.

The specific properties that make walking effective in the management and prevention of diabetes are:

- Walking for at least 5–10 minutes after a meal can help balance blood sugars.
- Often, being overweight can be an issue with diabetics, so walking with additional elements of fitness (see Chapter 4) can be a gentle

but effective way to lose weight. As you increase your exercise levels, using fitness poles (see page 89) also reduces strain on the knees, hips and feet. Complications with the feet are common with this condition and can impact on walking.

- Walking is something that can be done anywhere, is affordable and does not require specific exercise clothing, so is easier to include into a busy schedule and manage around food and drug regimes.
- Walking downhill is proven to use muscles in a way that can reduce blood sugar levels. However, uphill walking has other great benefits, such as building lean tissue and boosting metabolism, so unless you live by a ski lift it makes sense to do both!
- Walking can enable more mindful activities than other forms of exercise (see Chapter 2). Studies show that when people added some meditation via a mantra to a 12-week walking programme, they gained improvements in long-term blood sugar control, and reduction in stress hormones and arterial stiffness, when compared to those who walked without meditating.

CASE STUDY: DENIS COLLEN

Denis, who was diagnosed with type 2 diabetes in 2020, had always struggled with fitness.

'As part of my management plan I was advised to reduce my intake of carbs and exercise regularly, but I had never managed to include exercise regularly in my regime. I joined a health walking group and tried using poles too. Now I embrace the commitment to walk six days a week, and it provides exercise and mental wellbeing through being outdoors, plus valuable social connections. My wife and I both trained as walking instructors so we could share the benefits with others.'

Hip and knee pain or replacement

Upper-body joint pain is limiting in so many ways and often causes other conditions, due to the forced inactivity. It helps if those waiting for operations can stay as active as possible and, of course, walking with fitness poles can be a good aid in that regard.

I also advise a structured rehabilitation process following joint replacements. This should start with the exercises provided by the local physiotherapy team (which are essential), before graduating to walking indoors, using poles and building up steps.

The key is not to do too much too soon and to avoid activities that involve too much weight bearing, excessive bending, twisting, jumping or running, where all the bodyweight goes on to each leg in turn. The elements of fitness to include in your walking are CV for weight management, plus flexibility and strength exercises.

CASE STUDY: MALCOLM VINER

Malcolm explains how using poles and being part of a group helped his recovery after a hip replacement.

'After years of slowing down and doing less walking due to the pain of an arthritic hip, I had a new one fitted seven years ago. Once I had recovered from the surgery, I really wanted to get fit and mobile once more, and my specialist mentioned using poles. I tried a taster session and then enrolled in a course. I could immediately see the benefits as walking over varied terrain became easier and faster, so my stamina improved and steep hills were no longer something to dread on long walks. The regular and very varied walks available have meant seeing amazing parts of the countryside and meeting lots of lovely people.'

Menopause

This life phase can be debilitating for women as body changes can cause weight gain, mood swings, exhaustion and a host of other issues. I have worked closely with a menopause advice group set up by award-winning dietician Nigel Denby, whose plan uses walking and healthy eating to improve symptoms. While in many instances HRT or other interventions may be advised, I saw huge improvements in women who increased their steps and added total body walking principles to their daily lives over a 12-week 'back to basics' programme. I was heartened to hear how a daily walk became much more than their exercise, because of the positive effect it had on their mood and the time it gave them to themselves.

The key elements of fitness to include in a walking plan would be CV for weight management, and strength to help with toning and metabolism/weight. Being kind to yourself is also important, so make at least one walk a week about taking time to enjoy being out and in nature, with maybe some mindful yoga added in.

Living with excess weight

Weight management is not always easy and once weight reaches a certain point it begins to affect your ability to exercise, and therefore help to reduce it. Even walking can cause discomfort initially, with lower joint pain, chafing and lack of conditioning, but a managed walking programme using fitness poles can be effective and the poles increase calorie-burning, too.

It takes a lot of confidence to get started and I believe that if every step is a rewarding experience the process of walking is more likely to be effective in the longer term. Building in the joy of connecting with nature and some fun daily inspirations can make all the difference, while adding in strength exercises to your walking can also help to speed up weight loss due to the effects on your metabolism. Take things slowly then build in bursts of CV exercise, which you can increase as you get fitter.

High blood pressure

Regular exercise and maintaining a healthy weight are key ways to lower blood pressure, and walking is one of the best ways to start doing this. I advise brisk walking or changing the pace (see page 53) and mixing up walks, from short, faster bursts for 10 minutes to longer walks over trickier terrain.

It is important that those with hypertension attend regular blood pressure checks with their doctor and take medication, if prescribed. It's also a good idea to notify your doctor if you start a total body walking plan (see the Appendix). Once the exercise benefits begin to show, it might even be possible to gradually reduce your medication (under medical supervision, of course).

Parkinson's or balance conditions

It is difficult to give advice for progressive conditions that present in several ways. However, I have worked with many conditions and found that, in the early stages, brisk walking and using fitness poles have made a huge difference to fitness levels and management of the condition longer term.

Once freezing and tremors are present, I do advise the use of poles, but *never* those where the walker is strapped in. This can become a trip hazard for those with balance and mobility issues. Supervised exercise is also preferable, but there are lots of great groups that deliver walking sessions. The key elements of fitness to include are gentle strengthening, flexibility and balance exercises, plus concentrating on walking with good posture and purpose (see Chapter 1).

Fibromyalgia and rheumatic diseases

Conditions that cause pain, weakness and fatigue can make exercise difficult to manage, but a gentle programme of walking that includes all three elements of fitness (see Chapter 4) and becomes gradually more intense will work well. There is also a mood-boosting benefit to being outdoors – I have rarely seen gym programmes work as well as supportive walking in natural surroundings.

The key is to take things slowly and try to exercise when energy levels are at their highest, but always listen to pain signals and never push through pain or exhaustion. Using fitness poles can also help.

Cancer

Cancer treatment and recovery takes many forms, but just as walking can help to prevent many cancers, it is also one of the best ways to build back up to fitness and manage the often-debilitating treatment cycles involved.

I have seen great results with women with breast cancer, who find the arm movement that comes with walking – especially when using fitness poles – helps with lymphedema (swelling in the hands) and scar tissue management around mastectomy.

Over the years I have witnessed walking-based programmes improve the quality of life and confidence of those with a wide range of cancers, but I always advise people to consult specialists and trained exercise instructors.

It is important to take a holistic approach and take things slowly. I suggest you include stretching and light CV exercise in your walking, which you build up gradually, and gentle strengthening too. Some treatments affect balance, so it's a good idea to include some balance work as well.

CASE STUDY: CARO HAMES

Caro went through a year of treatment, including chemotherapy, radiotherapy and a lumpectomy for her breast cancer. She shared her wonder at how short walks with fitness poles gave her the confidence to plan a ski holiday:

'Honestly, I was laid to waste. I could hardly walk. I just hadn't got any energy and I lost my core, plus all my muscles in my legs. They all kind of got knotted – you get neuropathy as well with the chemo. I was making progress and then I had radiotherapy, which then again laid me to waste with fatigue.

'I was starting to walk again and my husband was training to be an instructor, and he persuaded me to walk with poles. It was just amazing. I could not believe it. I used to be a dancer in my earlier years so I've got quite a lot of cell memory in things like my core, but it was squidge – I mean totally squidge. When he showed me how to use the poles I honestly was only able to do 3 or 4km (1¾–2½ miles) at a time, probably max, but I just gradually built on it and by the time we went on holiday two months later, I had a bit of my core back and did some climbing mountains with him as well. They are fantastic for going up hills – honestly, just amazing!

'I was so chuffed with my progress and it was all to do with the poles, because I had stopped doing any other exercise. I am now back doing squats and lunges, because I want to go skiing in five months, and it looks like I'm going to be able to do that.

'I have to lose one week in every three, because when I've had the chemo, the first week I'm a bit low energy, but the second and the third week I'm out there with my poles. I just could not believe the difference to my core fitness – and I was getting bingo wings but they have gone now, too!'

Covid-19 or COPD

When breathlessness is an issue, it is difficult to motivate sufferers to begin to walk, but once they overcome that barrier and start slowly, walking can have massive benefits.

Obviously, lovely fresh air is a bonus, but those with breathing conditions need to be mindful if they are near traffic fumes, dusty areas and, of course, when pollen levels are high. Cold weather can affect our ability to exercise outdoors, too. For these reasons, in the past I have run walking sessions in air-conditioned shopping centres.

As some chronic obstructive pulmonary disease (COPD) sufferers also experience swollen legs and feet, walking poles are ideal. They help with posture and open the chest, which aids breathing. Walking with awareness of posture and natural movement, and gentle breathing exercises, can also help.

CASE STUDY: JULIA HOULTON

Julia found out how effective a gradual pole walking programme can be while recovering from Covid-19.

'I caught Covid-19 when skiing in France and ended up in hospital, where I spent six days on a ventilator, and then a week afterwards while the physiotherapists reminded me how to sit up, stand up and then walk.

'I was discharged home, equipped with a Zimmer frame on wheels, and was hardly able to stagger more than from the kerb to the front door. After a couple of weeks, I'd built up to walking for about 10 minutes a day.

'Anyway, the point of all this is that pushing the Zimmer frame caused both my arms to extend forwards to grip the handles. I then decided to try going out with my poles, and the benefits were immediate and considerable. Using the poles opens up my chest so I can breathe and walk at the same time. I've just come in from a 35-minute walk!

'I seriously don't think I'd be at this point yet without the poles. Being on a ventilator causes muscles to disappear – it's quite scary how fast they disappear – it's a slow job to build them back again.'

To reiterate, before you embark on a significant walking regime, do talk to your doctor and, if you can, a qualified exercise referral practitioner. Discuss your particular condition with them and how it could be improved by walking. Walking can be an extraordinarily powerful medicine.

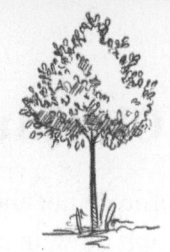

CHAPTER

8

WALK THIS WAY...
For correct kit and comfort

When you go for a walk, comfort is key and this chapter will help you to decide what food, drink, clothing (including what to wear on your feet), bags and other kit you will need, and how to prepare for going out.

The golden rule, of course, is to plan for the weather. Even a short walk can be uncomfortable if you get too wet, and there's simply no need for this, because good waterproof clothing is both lightweight and affordable. I know that I embrace walking in the rain, but if that causes you to get cold or develop blisters it could mean missing future walks – staying dry means you will love walking in any weather. Therefore, before heading out, it's a good idea to make it a habit to consider the following:

- How long will I be out?
- What is the weather likely to do in that time? (See page 146.)
- How much effort am I putting in today – is it a workout or a wander?

Getting thirsty or being hungry will spoil a good walk and, if you are exercising, impair your performance, so once you've answered the above questions, you'll be in a good position to make sensible decisions about what to take and what to wear.

Clothing

You do not always need to dress specifically for a walk. Obviously, we can and do walk in everyday clothing, from jeans to dresses, and that's why walking is a brilliant way to be more active. Walking should be integral to your daily life and not always a mission, so if you are comfortable and your footwear is suitable, you are good to go for an energising walk. However, once you start to consider upping the pace, increasing the distance or venturing further afield, it becomes more important to consider specialist clothing that can help keep you comfortable.

A lovely relaxing wander may simply require comfy clothing and a phone for safety. A short, fast blast relatively near to home requires minimal kit (although the effort level may dictate breathable clothing). But would I advocate minimal kit for fitness walking, longer hikes and walks in the wilds? Of course not. Then you may need spare layers, food and hydration.

Walking to work and changing your shoes when you get there or having a pair of trainers to change into for a lunchtime walk can be a great way to get your steps in, but it can get laborious if it involves a shower and a full clothing change. Get into the practice of being prepared. I have different walking kit for different scenarios, but it's all stored where I can grab what I need quickly. This is important because motivation can soon wane if you are searching for your socks or spending more time getting ready for a walk than actually out there enjoying it.

Layers

The one word I always start with when asked about clothing for walkers is *layers*. Even if you are dressed perfectly for the weather when you start a walk, your temperature is likely to change during it, even if the weather does not (which in itself is unlikely these days!). The concept has been used by hikers and outdoor workers for years – use thin layers that can be added or removed rather than a bulky coat, which once removed can be a burden.

This layering formula just involves thinking about what is close to your skin and what can be added or taken away according to the conditions and how you are feeling. The lighter the layers are, the more adaptable you become as you can carry them easily, giving you the option to add or remove them at will. I will explain each layer below so you can consider what might work for you.

BASE LAYER

You are likely to perspire when doing longer walks or pace or fitness exercises. Therefore, the layer next to your skin needs to be able to wick away this moisture, so you avoid feeling uncomfortable and chilling down. Breathable fabrics help to keep you dry and feel much nicer than a soaked T-shirt. However, many base layers are synthetic, so although they dry very quickly, they tend to smell after a while. I always opt for natural fabrics like merino or bamboo to have close to the skin. These seem to wash well and are comfy too.

MID LAYER

This is your warm insulating layer. Ideally it also needs to 'breathe'. Fleeces are a popular choice as you can get varying thicknesses from micro fleece to chunkier weave. All allow moisture to wick away and provide insulation.

On a dry day, these are often your outer layer. On wet or very windy days, they may be under a final layer that cuts out the worst of the weather, which makes a difference to the thickness required. I am a fan of the insulating gilet, which keeps the core warm but does not restrict movement.

OUTER LAYER

Once again, there are variations, from padded, insulated winter jackets to thin raincoats that just keep the water out or block the chill of the wind. The latter are great to pack on changeable days and are designed less for warmth. Most outdoor retailers now do three-in-one coats that are waterproof, but have a removeable mid layer – a great idea as a starting point. However, there are so many variables with jackets that over time it's good to have some staples to select from.

One item I have found invaluable is a fully waterproof cape with a hood. It can be put on quickly over any outfit and a backpack as it has poppers on the sides. In squalls I have even crouched down and used it almost as a tent! Lightweight and versatile, it's a must-have in my pack.

Underwear

A word about underwear if you intend to do long day hikes or push yourself with some fitness walking exercises. Wearing sports-specific undergarments will help with comfort level and the same rules as base layers apply when it comes to fabrics. It is important that underwear is not too tight.

SPORTS BRAS

Walkers with breasts need to support them, both for comfort and to avoid damage if doing any bouncy moves. Breasts are held up by connective tissue called the Cooper's ligaments which, unlike muscles, cannot be restored once damaged. Sports bras come with wider supportive straps, mesh panels for breathability and added support for the breasts. As they are typically quick drying, you can stay comfortable and dry them overnight after washing.

SOCKS

Socks are more important than many people realise. They should wick the moisture away from your feet and protect them from friction to prevent blisters. Good walking socks should be padded in certain areas like the toe box and back of the heel. There are also some technical ranges that provide cross support for ankles and mesh panels to let the heat out.

The key is that socks must fit well. Whether you opt for the old-style woolly socks or sportier walking models, if they do not fit snugly you will be liable to develop blisters. If there is too much room your feet can slide around, causing the socks to bunch, which is uncomfortable and will cause pressure points.

I advise spending as much as you can afford on walking socks, because cheaper ones never last and are often not breathable, so feet overheat and get damp. This is another cause of blisters and will also result in bacteria, which can lead to athlete's foot and unpleasant odours. A good rule of thumb is to look for the padding and whether the socks are breathable. Opting for natural fabrics is ideal, too, although I am personally not a fan of woollen socks close to the skin.

Clothing accessories

There are lots of walking accessories that can help you to regulate temperature and stay comfortable.

HEADWEAR FOR WARMER DAYS

It is essential to protect the head, neck and face from the sun. Many caps are breathable with mesh panels, UV protection and even built-in neck panels. Lightweight caps and visors shield the eyes and can serve to keep the hair under control, too. This is a bonus if you are exercising or out on a windy day.

For more relaxed walking, there is a multitude of wide-brimmed hats to choose from, with my favourite being those that scrunch up easily when not in use. Australian-style outback hats are great – minus the corks, of course. These days, you can get integral insect repellent or mesh drop-downs to ward off midges instead.

HEADWEAR FOR COLDER DAYS

You will often be warned about how much heat is lost from the head, but typically this is because it is the only part of us that is not covered with clothing. Pop a hat on and you are insulating yourself fully from the cold. Choose from the traditional woollen beanie or bobble hat, or go more technical with waterproofing as well. In wet weather, you may need the latter if you don't have a hood to pull up over your hat, because wool is not ideal when wet and heavy.

TIP

You can get caps and hats that have fluorescent panels or torches built into them. These are great when out at night or in fog.

NECKWEAR

Covering your neck provides exceptional warmth on colder days, but can also protect against heat and the sun in summer. The neck tube or buff is something I always have in my pack, because they are lightweight and adaptable. You can turn them into headbands or hats, or simply pop them around your neck to keep the heat in. On hot days, they are great soaked in cold water to keep you cool. If you intend to walk in really hot climates, you can get a 'Lawrence of Arabia'-style combination of hat and neck shield.

Footwear

What constitutes a good pair of shoes for walking is a personal choice that can vary from person to person. Different walkers have different gaits and style preferences. While some prefer low-rise walking trainers or barefoot shoes, others favour stout, ankle-supporting walking boots. With a wealth of footwear choices available, when it comes to walking shoes, I am going to advise you what *not* to wear, before looking at the best types of footwear to try, so you can walk in optimum comfort.

My first no-no is the good old wellington boot. I know there are trendier, softer ones available these days, which are easy to pull on and which protect against mud, *but* they are simply not designed for walking with good posture (unless you opt for expensive ranges designed for shooting). Many wellies have a small, hard heel section that does not allow the foot to roll naturally (see page 70) and they often don't have any cushioning. They tend to not hold the feet snugly, causing them to move around inside the boots. This can be countered with thick socks, but I prefer a laced-up shoe that can be fitted more accurately. If you intend to walk for fitness, wellies are definitely not recommended.

Leather walking boots have made a comeback recently and, while I applaud the natural material and attention to detail on the better ones, I do feel many are too heavy and inflexible to provide the natural gait and connection I like to have with the ground. Some tend to restrict the mobility of the foot, causing a solid, flat-footed plant, which is often due to inflexible soles.

Lightweight walking boots

Lightweight, waterproof and breathable boots (typically walking footwear that encases the ankle) are more flexible and certainly advisable when fitness walking. These are made by most outdoor and running shoe manufacturers. Opt for waterproof and breathable boots (fabrics such as Gore-Tex™ or similar) if you can afford it, because wet feet are uncomfortable and prone to blisters. Boot styles do provide more ankle stability, but I only find this becomes necessary if you intend to hike on very gnarly terrain or have a weakness in the ankles or lower legs.

Mid shoes, trainers and trail shoes

'Mid shoes' are essentially trainers with greater ankle support – known as low rise – or you can opt for the more natural feel of lower, less-supportive trainers and trail shoes. The soles need to match the type of walking you do regularly, though. There is no need for super-grippy, tyre-like tracks if you walk on grassy paths or pavements, but if you venture into rocky terrain these are essential.

It's important to invest in good-quality walking shoes if you can; the feet are very complex and have a huge job to do, so look after them. There are specific makes of walking shoes designed to encourage good heel strike and foot roll, too. The GRUBS Discover™ walking shoe has what they call RollinGait™' technology, while Skechers produce their GOWalk™ shoes designed for both city and urban trails. Ecco has also put a lot of research and design into their walking shoes, which certainly do provide excellent comfort.

If you notice that over time your trainers and shoes tend to lean towards the centre or outer edge, you might want to get your gait analysed before building up your miles. A good podiatrist will provide orthotics that can correct foot problems and help you avoid knee, hip and back issues.

'Healthy feet can hear the very heart of the earth' – Sitting Bull, Sioux warrior

Barefoot shoes

Barefoot (or minimal) shoes are designed to mirror the natural shape of feet and how they connect with the ground. Brands like Vivobarefoot and Xero Shoes have thin soles and wider toe boxes to allow the spread of the toes when walking. They do feel natural and lightweight, but take some getting used to. Nothing replaces the connection you get with the ground when actually barefoot, though (see page 152).

Look for 'hiking, walking and trail shoes' to find the weight and flexibility that suits you. Fit and comfort are far more important than the look of shoes, so it is important to take your time when choosing them. Try them on later in the day when your feet are hotter and have been taking your weight, always with the socks you would normally wear when walking. Feel for tightness at the toes and slipping at the heel, bending the shoe with your foot in it to check this.

Bags

If your walk is long enough to require extra clothing and some food, the most comfortable way to carry it is via a backpack, which distributes the weight and allows you to move easily. If you are walking for fitness or using poles, you will need to choose a smaller backpack or cross-body bag to allow for a good arm swing.

Backpacks

Backpacks are typically sold by their capacity in litres. A small pack for your daily walks could be 10 or 15 litres. If you will be out all day, your pack size would ideally be around 25–30 litres, as you may want food, water and more safety items. In colder weather you may need to up this to allow room to carry extra warm layers. Choose packs with padded shoulders, extra pockets and expandable areas, in case you remove more layers.

Always look for waist and chest straps, which stop the bag bouncing as you walk. As your back is likely to get warm when you walk, it is good to check for mesh or breathable fabrics on the back of the bag too – some even hold the pack away from you, allowing air to flow through. Women need to select packs designed to adjust around the chest area or opt for those specifically made for their shape.

FITTING A BACKPACK

When trying out backpacks, always pop some weight into them and then loosen all the straps. Make sure the waist belt or strap fits nicely first and then adjust the shoulder straps. They should fit well with no gaps. Finally, adjust the chest strap to hold the pack in place. Try bending, stretching and jumping a bit to test for comfort – you will be glad you did.

Waist packs

Waist packs are great for walking as they keep the back clear and so reduce that sweaty feeling. You can get well-fitted ones that just carry the essentials and a water bottle in a secure holder. These are great for workout walks and are popular with pole users as they do not restrict the arms. There are larger ones available that will also hold a layer of clothing, or some snacks, but if they are too big these can bounce around a bit.

Cross-body bags

For those who don't want to embrace the backpack or hiker look, there are lots of cross-body bags that enable you to walk freely and keep your hands free for touching, arm movements and so on. The sportier ones, like the Osprey Daylite Sling, are also well fitted and work for faster walking and workouts too. Cross-body bags can be worn on the front or back; if they are front-facing they are ideal for accessing phones for listening to podcasts or music.

TIP

Even those who like to walk with minimal kit invariably have a phone, so phone armbands can be useful, too.

What to carry

Some walkers seem to take everything they might conceivably need on *every* walk, while others, like me, prefer to travel light, but still have the essentials to hand according to the effort level, location and weather.

If I am going for a short, mindful stroll, I take a cross-body bag with phone, keys and perhaps a foraging pouch (see page 134). If I intend to push the pace, but am near to home (negating the need for extra layers), I will upgrade to a waist pack with water bottle. On a cold day, longer walks or fitness walks, I take a 15-litre backpack, because a first-aid kit, layers and food could be required, especially if I am going out into wilder areas.

Let's lay out the kit essentials, so you can make an instant decision as to what you might need on each walk you undertake.

Phone

You should *always* carry a fully charged mobile phone (or a means of contact) with you, because not only might you trip or fall, but you may take a wrong turn or come across somebody else in trouble. See page 137 for advice on safety.

You may also want it to track your route, access podcasts, identify plants and even use a timer to count your workout moves! See page 143 for recommended apps.

> **TIP**
>
> It's worth investing in a waterproof mobile phone case.

First-aid kit

I think there's merit in having a mini first-aid kit, containing a couple of plasters and a foil blanket, with you on most walks. There are envelope-style ones available, which take up little space and are lightweight. I also carry a calendula cuts and grazes spray, which is great for bramble incidents.

For longer walks, a walkers' first-aid kit that opens out and has everything you need to deal with cuts, sprains and other injuries is ideal. Blister plasters are always a good idea, although prevention is better than cure, so if you tend to get blisters it might be worth looking up the PelliTec® pads, which go into your shoes at friction points.

Water

If you are exerting yourself on a short walk or out for over an hour you should carry water – or at least know where you can access clean water en route. Never wait until you are thirsty, as this can affect both your health and your performance. Likewise, never venture out in hot weather without adequate water supplies or the knowledge of where you can fill up.

Hydration is not simply about staving off thirst: being dehydrated increases the risk of strokes and other serious conditions, and exacerbates the symptoms of other conditions. If you have had achy joints recently, for instance, it could be related to lack of hydration. Similarly, if you are finding you have no energy, top up your water level instead of reaching for a snack.

It is advisable to drink before a walk, every 20 minutes or so when walking and at the end of a walk, too. If you are losing a lot of water due to sweating on an endurance hike or similar, it's a good idea to have some electrolyte tablets with you as you will be losing essential minerals, not just water.

Check out the best way to comfortably carry the water you need for the walk you have planned and take time to chill it before your walk. Metal water bottles are not only great for the planet, but they also keep water nice and cool if you put them in the fridge overnight and pop ice cubes in before you leave. There are also great backpacks with integral 'bladders', but they are quite tricky to keep clean. Whichever way you choose to carry it water is pretty heavy (0.9kg/2lb per 1 litre/1¾ pints) and we need about 2 litres (3½ pints) a day to stay hydrated – more when walking briskly or in hot weather.

If you are out in wilder locations, use a water filtration bottle that can purify water. I love the Water-to-Go™ bottle, which is not only great for everyday use as it filters tap water, but also when walking abroad, especially where water supplies may be less reliable.

Note: Filtration will not kill all viruses, so if walking wild you may need to take a stove to boil water or explore sanitisation tablets.

If, like me, you like warm drinks, take a small carry flask with you. Fill it with your favourite beverage or just take hot water and indulge in what nature provides (see page 195). If you get into the tea infusion idea, you can invest in an infusion flask, which has a filter for your chosen leaves and flowers. Alternatively, make up tea bags with dried mint, lemon balm or dandelions from the garden to pop in your backpack. There are some lovely eco bamboo infuser flasks available, which are equally suitable for home and work.

Cooling towel

A real game-changer on hot days, these towels have special cells that store water and feel freezing cold to touch when exposed to air. Many come in special holders to attach to your backpack. Choose whether to dampen your towel at home or en route, then simply swing in the air for a delicious freezing cold wrap to press on your face or around your neck when the going gets hot. Cooling towels are also good for sprains.

Sunscreen and sunglasses

Your skin and eyes are as important as every other organ in your body, so don't expose them to too much direct sunlight. Use sunscreen before going out for a walk and regularly on any areas that are uncovered, even on duller days. Always have some in your pack for longer walks.

Pop on some sunglasses to protect your eyes from damage. Many eye conditions, such as cataracts, age-related macular degeneration and skin cancer, can be exacerbated by exposure to UV rays. On windy days, sunglasses also protect your eyes from dust, pollen and sand. In snowy conditions, the glare from the whiteness can cause snow blindness too.

Whistle or personal alarm

If you are lost and trying to alert others to your whereabouts, a whistle can be a great help. Personal alarms can make you feel safer in some locations.

Tick remover

Tick bites can cause Lyme disease (see page 139). A tick remover takes up little space, but could be invaluable. I use a credit-card sized one that has hooks for different-sized ticks and a magnifying glass so you can see what you are doing.

Food

Being hungry will spoil a good walk and, if you're exercising, impair your performance. It is important to have a few staples to hand which are high energy, healthy and easy to carry; ideally items that can stay in the pack in case they are needed in an emergency, but are a delicious treat on any stop.

Unsurprisingly, trail mix is a great option. Typically, a mix of dried fruit, nuts and granola, it helps with energy levels, does not melt and can be home-made or shop bought. Similarly, energy balls or bars are a good choice. It's good practice to keep an energy gel pouch in your larger pack in case you get injured, stranded or come across somebody else in need of nutrition.

Power bites

Lucie, a nutritionist, gave me this recipe and it's a winner. Use these energy balls for walking or to counteract that mid-afternoon dip. You can play around with other dried fruits of your choice and substitute the pecan nuts for walnuts, cashews or hazelnuts, if you wish. If you use hard dates, they will be more difficult to blend and may require soaking.

Ingredients

325g (1½ cups) Medjool or soft stoned dates

- 35g (⅓ cup) pecan nuts
- 1 tbsp peanut butter (smooth or crunchy)
- 1 tbsp cocoa powder
- ¼ tsp ground cinnamon

Method

Blend everything together in a blender until smooth and then work into bite-sized balls with your hands. Store in the fridge or freezer.

Extras to carry for nature connection

If you get into the nature connection invitations (see page 174), you might want to pack the following items too.

SOFT SEAT PAD

Having a comfortable, portable seat will allow you to sit for longer periods among the trees and flowers. Most outdoor stores have great fold-up or blow-up options.

JEWELLER'S MAGNIFIER OR LOUPE

When looking closely at things, a magnifying glass can make a moment in nature magical. They are easy to purchase online and take up little room in your pack.

FORAGING POUCH

I always make sure I have a foraging pouch, in case I see something to gather (with permission, of course). They fit on to your waist packs and expand as you fill them, but fold up small when not in use. The reuseable mesh bags that you put your supermarket veg in will do the same job.

TIP

If you are spending time with wildlife, don't forget to take birdseed or seed bombs to entice them in.

WILDLIFE GUIDEBOOKS

There's nothing more frustrating than spotting something wonderful, but being unable to identify it. Apps are great, but using a phone can remove that connection to nature. Lightweight wildlife guides or mini books still get my vote – they are old school but easy to use. I still have the tiny books about trees and birds I had as a child, but you can also get wild ID field guides that are intended for use outdoors. The Field Studies Council produces guides for education, but also has some that are ideal for walkers.

NOTEBOOK

I have my best ideas when walking and, if I am not in the mood to get my phone out to dictate, love to jot them down in a notebook. Of course, many of those ideas come to me when the weather is wet, so I now use waterproof notepads. If you are a notetaker or sketcher, these are brilliant and, while there are quite a few brands available now, for years I have used the Rite in the Rain® ones developed for the US military.

Extras to carry for fitness and performance

To turn a stroll into a workout walk, it is useful to pack some basic strength equipment, such as exercise resistance bands, weighted balls or neoprene sand bag weights. It is also well worth investing in a pair of fitness poles (see page Chapter 4).

EXERCISE RESISTANCE BANDS

All types of bands and details of the most common exercises they are used for can be found on the internet. Learn and practise at home before taking them out with you, to make sure you are getting it right.

There are four main types of resistance bands that work well for walking workouts:

1 **Looped vinyl bands:** Often sold in a pack of different resistance strengths, these loops enable you to perform several lower- and upper-body exercises. They are lightweight and take up little space in your pack.
2 **Cut-to-length or straight vinyl bands:** Again, these come in different resistance levels, often reflected by colour (no two brands use the same colour codes, so be aware). Use these to perform the same exercises as with loops. Increase the resistance by shortening the section of the band you are pulling against.
3 **Thicker fabric leg bands:** These bands are designed to fit around the legs to add resistance and effectiveness to squats and lunges. They are typically made from a non-slip fabric material and are about 10–12.5cm (4–5in) deep to ensure they do not roll up or cut into the flesh.
4 **Bands with a handle at each end:** Handles make the grip easier. They can be used for a multitude of exercises, including making bicep curls more comfortable (see page 109). It is harder to shorten them to increase resistance, though.

WEIGHTED BALLS AND NEOPRENE SANDBAG WEIGHTS

These are great for performing resistance exercises on the go. Both will also add weight to your backpack for a workout walk, but make sure you stop the weight from bouncing around and fit your pack properly. Weighted balls come in different sizes, but I would suggest getting ones that fit into one hand easily, because they are more versatile. Chi balls are also great for coordination and balance exercises, and are lighter and deflate, so they can be carried easily.

TOTAL BODY OR FITNESS WALKING POLES

If you want to walk with poles, see Chapter 4 for an understanding of fitness poles and how they adjust, because this will help you determine the typical components or spares you may need. I do not advocate using one walking pole only.

Rubber ferrules or 'paws', designed for use on hard surfaces, usually come with good-quality poles. They provide a nice silent grip and less-jarring vibration than the tungsten tips which are for use on softer terrain. It's a good idea to carry spares if you do walk on hard surfaces or the tapping sound can spoil your walk!

Pole adjustment

Walking poles may be fixed in length or adjustable for height (I recommend the latter). Some are telescopic and break down into three sections, which is useful if you are travelling or wish to pop them into a backpack. Bear in mind that this will increase vibration, so for regular users a two-part pole that adjusts mid shaft will be more comfortable.

Some poles adjust with a simple twist-lock function, which is opened and shut by twisting the top and bottom of the pole shaft in different directions – hold the poles horizontally in front of you with one hand on each section. Once you reach the desired height, simply twist each section back the other way to tighten at that height.

Other poles have a clip lock, which needs to be opened to facilitate the height adjustment. With these it is important the clip is kept nice and tight. Guides to help with this are available on the WALX website .

Extras to carry for dog owners

If you like to have your companion with you on walks, always take a lead in case of grazing animals and other dangers. All animals can be unpredictable, even the most well-trained of dogs. You might also like to explore waist harnesses that enable the dog to stay attached, but keep your hands free for foraging, exercising and using poles. The best ones are designed for canicross, a sport where you run with your dog.

Finally, as every dog lover knows, you need some treats and compostable poo bags. It may seem madness to pick up dog poo when there are piles of cow pats in a field, but please do, as dogs carry germs and diseases that can harm other species. If you are not a fan of carrying your steaming bags, invest in a scented zip-up container like a Dicky Bag, which clips on to your belt or the dog's lead. Never fall into the trap of leaving the bag to pick up on your way home – the amount of bags hanging in trees is testament to the fact that people rarely remember to do so.

Staying safe on a walk

Some of the information earlier in this chapter (see page 129) touches on items that may help you to stay safe, but I think this important topic also warrants a more detailed run-through.

Stay connected

I mentioned always having a phone with you (see page 130) and, as much as I like a digital detox, I stand by this. I have heard about incidents happening to walkers on all types of walks, from short local strolls to an ascent of a mountain peak. Risks in urban parks may differ from those in open countryside, but I have heard of people encountering stags in city parks and being mugged on a leafy rural path. Luckily both are rare and walking is a very safe activity, but it pays to stay connected just in case. Why risk being unable to get help or to notify somebody of your whereabouts?

It is a good idea to load your ICE (in case of emergency) information into your phone – the contact(s) that you would want to be notified should you be hurt or unwell – and any information regarding medication or allergies. iPhone users can load this via the Health app; on Android phones it tends to be under Settings or the Personal Safety app. Both types of phone also have an SOS procedure – for how to use this search for your phone model on the internet.

You may also want to use your phone to track your route, but a word of warning here. You can share with friends or family, so they know where you are (see page 144), but do not share this publicly via apps.

Also, be careful when wearing earphones. If what you're listening to is too loud, you may not be able to hear traffic, anyone approaching you from behind or warnings.

Know where you are

If you intend to go for long hikes or treks in wilder places where the signal could be poor, you may want to explore a GPS messenger, such as the Garmin inReach®. This transfers from cellular mobile phone to GPS if you need to send a message or get help when out of range of the phone network.

Adding the what3words app to your phone is worthwhile, too, especially if you are going into wilder areas, because it helps you to tell others where you are and direct emergency services anywhere in the world. The what3words website explains how to use it.

In case of an incident, you might also want to load an app that can help you to locate the nearest defibrillator.

Protect yourself from bites and stings

The best way to avoid bites and stings is to cover up in high-risk areas, and to use sprays and bracelets to put insects off. Try to use natural deterrents made from plant oils such as citronella and reapply regularly.

Wear long trousers when walking through long grasses, make sure you have sleeves if your route takes you through taller vegetation, and seek out hats with nets for midge-infested areas. It might seem like overkill, but tick bites need to be avoided at all costs and mosquito bites are pretty unpleasant, too.

Lyme disease

This bacterial infection can cause long-term debilitation and is spread by infected ticks. These nasty critters lurk in long grasses and bracken, and jump on to their next host as they walk by. Attracted by the warmth and blood, they latch on and feed until they drop off.

Before you set out, check whether you are walking in a high-risk area for ticks – there are online maps that will tell you this – and take the precautions above. If you do find a tick, remove it immediately with a proper tick remover (see page 132). Do not burn it with a match.

While most bites will just result in an itch, if you are unlucky and the tick infects you with Lyme disease you may develop a rash around the bite (which can resemble a bullseye) and could become ill with flu-like symptoms. Always seek medical advice if either of these occur or you experience other concerns following a bite. For more information see the Lyme Disease UK website (see page 213).

Be aware of other path users

In parks, the paths could be used by runners, cyclists, skateboarders (if allowed) and people with prams. It is important to be polite when overtaking and careful if using fitness poles, so you don't trip anybody up.

Make sure you are visible by wearing brighter clothing on dull, misty and darker days, and headtorches or flashing lights if appropriate. On country lanes, visibility is key – even on brighter days – as traffic may not be expecting walkers.

DOGS

Dogs are increasingly popular and not all owners have full control over their pets. Always slow down and avoid sudden movements when you encounter an unsupervised dog. Some are spooked by poles or strange or fast movements, such as fitness exercises. Some dog owners use extending leads, so check for those to avoid trips.

HORSES AND GRAZING ANIMALS

On footpaths, you may encounter horses or even grazing animals. Horses also get spooked by poles and sudden movement, so always slow down and stay calm in their presence.

Cows are typically docile, but if they have calves with them they can be protective and aggressive, particularly if you are walking with a dog. Always let your dog off a lead so it can run to safety if they do begin to gather. If you're walking without a dog and receive too much attention, try to stay calm and assertive when walking away. Raise your hands and calmly say 'woah' if they follow.

Bulls from recognised dairy stock should never be in fields with footpaths running through them, while on occasion some lesser-known breeds (thought to be less aggressive) could be. Younger bulls may also be in with mothers and calves, and tend to have no interest in walkers unless they present a perceived risk. Skirt round or take a detour, if possible, and remain calm, always moving slowly.

Sheep and lambs are generally not concerned by walkers, but avoid spooking them, especially if ewes are pregnant or have become separated from their lambs.

Staying safe in bad weather

Although I advocate walking in all weathers, I would advise caution about starting a walk if there is a yellow weather warning in your area. This may be for excessive heat, heavy snow, floods or high winds. Use your weather app and TV forecasts (see page 143) to make sure you know what could be coming your way.

STORMS

If you are caught out in thunder, move away from tall, isolated structures like trees, which may conduct the lightning strike. Let go of any walking poles or metal items and stay as close to the ground as possible. A crouching position is best, tucking your hands and head into your knees in order to minimise contact with the ground. Never lie down on the ground as that means a larger surface area of your body will be exposed.

Note: If your hair stands on end, you are very close to the storm and must take up the crouch position immediately.

SNOW AND ICE

Snowfall can be magical, even exhilarating, to walk in, but in windy conditions be aware of sudden drifts, which can block paths and make walking difficult. If venturing out in snowy conditions, always make sure you are dressed appropriately and have emergency provisions. A pair of studded ice cleats over your shoe soles will make all the difference if you need to walk in icy conditions. Fitness poles can help, too.

Be aware that while powdery snow is lovely, it becomes much heavier if wet, and ice can form underneath if it has started to melt and then frozen again. Walking on hard, icy ground is treacherous, so try to stick to grassy areas and avoid icy puddles, even though they are fun to crack.

In this chapter I've talked about what to take with you and how to stay safe. I have given you advice to cover every eventuality – at least, every eventuality I can think of! – so in conclusion, all I can say is, once again, whatever kind of walk it is and wherever you're going, be prepared!

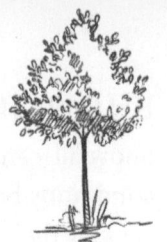

9

WALK THIS WAY...
To stay motivated

These days our lives are very busy and this can impact on the time we have available for ourselves and for exercise. Even when we do establish a routine that includes exercise, unexpected events can mean we lapse and that tends to make it even harder to get back into the routine. Holidays, while refreshing, can break a routine, as can sickness, work and family commitments. However, I have studied behaviour change in relation to exercise and know that the likelihood of adhering to any exercise regime can be increased by the following three factors:

1. **Results:** If you can see exercise working, you are more likely to keep doing it.
2. **Enjoyment:** If it's fun-filled and full of variety, you are less likely to get bored with exercise.
3. **Sociality:** Exercising with others is a powerful motivator.

These are the foundation blocks of total body walking, and there are plenty of tools and tips that relate to these and can help you in this chapter. Flick through and see what could work for you.

1. Results

It is important to see and feel results from any exercise regime, and walking is no different. Follow these steps to set yourself goals and challenges, add progression to your workouts and learn how to track your workouts and achievements. When you achieve results, remind yourself of how far you've come and reward yourself– which we can sometimes forget to do. Practise taking time to check in with yourself and notice the small things. Are you sleeping better? Do you have more energy than before? Or are you simply walking faster or feeling more stable on your feet? Congratulate yourself for every improvement – every good result will lead to another!

Set yourself a goal

Whether your challenge is to walk a set amount of miles in a set time or to increase your speed, simple goals can help and you will be surprised at how good it feels when you achieve them. Check out the daily inspirations (see Chapter 10) for ideas, which can range from Munro bagging (see page 197) to walking a long-distance path (see page 158).

Have a mantra and keep repeating it if times get tough. It could be simple – 'I will fit into those trousers' – or more extreme – 'I will climb Ben Nevis.' Either way, say it, repeat it and you will *do* it. Commit to entering a challenge event or charity walk that you need to build up towards. Tell people about it and you will not want to fail.

Use apps and websites to stay on track

Use route-finding, map and tracking apps to count and record your progress. Some have communities where you can share routes and measure your time for certain walks against others. Others have challenges where you can record cumulative miles or sign up to a virtual trek across the Andes or similar. During the Covid-19 lockdowns, these helped walkers stay connected as well as motivated.

WALKING WEBSITES OR APPS TO HELP WITH DAILY INSPIRATIONS, ROUTES AND COMMUNITIES

- **WALX** (walx.co.uk): For online courses and sessions, groups, tuition and community.
- **Ramblers** (www.ramblers.org.uk): A website with information, groups and regional led walks.
- **The Long Distance Walkers Association** (ldwa.org.uk): For a database of paths, organised groups and challenge events.

- **NHS Active 10** (www.nhs.uk/better-health/get-active): A great tracker app that can help you build daily activity levels.
- **GO Jauntly** (gojauntly.com): An urban-based app with routes and a nature notes feature.
- **World Walking** (worldwalking.org): This website provides routes all over the world for you to embark on virtually.
- **Walkopedia** (www.walkopedia.net): Information and routes to help you plan treks and walks around the globe.
- **American Hiking** (americanhiking.org): Great resource for finding trails in the US, plus getting involved in protecting them via volunteering.
- **Trail Hiking Australia** (trailhiking.com.au): Resources for planning to walk a trail in Australia plus a community and advice on kit etc.
- **WALX Taiwan** (walx.tw): Total body walking tuition, regular group walks plus trips and walking tours in Taiwan.

ROUTE FINDING, MAP AND TRACKING APPS

Many of these started with one function, such as route planning or mileage tracking, but have morphed into offering many of the same features:

- **Endomondo** (endomondo.com): A route tracking and sharing app for runners walkers and cyclists.
- **Strava** (strava.com): A community and fitness tracking app where hikers, runners and cyclists share routes and track progress.
- **MapMyWalk** (mapmywalk.com): A great app for storing routes you have walked and tracking your milage, speed and so on.
- **AllTrails** (alltrails.com). Brilliant for finding walks near you and following routes.
- **Outdooractive** (outdooractive.com): Great for any activity outdoors, maps routes and community.
- **Ordnance Survey** (ordnancesurvey.co.uk). A bank of UK-based maps and walks.
- **Fitbit**: More about mileage, steps and exercise.
- **Apple and Garmin watches**: Combine all the above.

'The best way to get started is to quit talking and begin doing' – Walt Disney

Keep a journal

If you don't want to use a phone to track your progress, writing a record of each walk in a journal is equally effective. Record anything you feel is relevant:

- Where you walked
- Distance
- Time taken
- Pace
- Elements of fitness used (see Chapter 4)
- Daily inspirations used (see Chapter 10)
- Time of day
- Type of terrain
- How you felt before and after

Add progression

If you do not add progression to your programme, you may start to wonder if the time and effort are worth it. When you're new to walking, it's common to notice increased energy, weight loss and feelings of joy, but the results begin to slow if you don't consciously add in extra bursts of speed, miles, hills or exercise elements that increase the intensity. This is known as the plateau effect and it's why it can help to join a group with a leader who pushes you a little harder than you might be inclined to go if left to your own devices.

You can just count your repetitions for most exercises (see page 60), but sometimes you might want to do set times of a particular exercise and then have a designated rest time before doing it again.

EXERCISE TIMER APPS FOR INTERVALS OR TIMING WORKOUT PACE EXERCISES

The following are used by a lot of total body walking instructors to help sessions flow and make sure people work hard enough. I've suggested some but have a look at your app store for what is available.

- **HITT Timer:** Sounds to let you know when it's time to start and rest.
- **Speaking Timer:** Perfect for exercise on the move, as it speaks to you.
- **Time Rise:** An old-fashioned visual egg timer.

2. Enjoyment

If you enjoy an exercise and it releases some of those all-important feel-good endorphins, you will want to do it time and time again. You can add an extra level of fun and indulgence to your daily walk by being mindful, studying the nature around you, listening to music, and adding variety and progression to your walks. The daily inspirations (see Chapter 10) are designed to provide that variety, give you ideas to relieve boredom and information to keep you engaged. Flick through and jot down the ones that will work for you in the coming weeks.

Mix and match

Add variety and progression to your regular walks (for example, make things slightly harder each week) to keep things fresh while ensuring continual results. If you keep doing the same walks or workouts at the same intensity, you will stop noticing results and you'll get bored. Think about trying different routes and terrains if you tend to go the same way every day.

Jazz it up

If you are motivated by music, make a walking playlist. This is especially useful if the noise where you walk is not full of birdsong or rustling leaves. Music is known to distract you from the sense that you're making an effort, so it can help when pushing yourself harder on pace exercises, too.

Be prepared for the weather

There's nothing less enjoyable than being unprepared when walking. Getting cold and wet is not only uncomfortable and potentially dangerous, but it will also demotivate you. Avoid it at all costs by having the correct clothing and checking the weather forecasts before you set out. I like AccuWeather. Wherever you are in the world it shows the weather in your area in real time, so you can watch the fronts coming in and see what's happening in the next hour or so.

Study the world around you

Have fun identifying the plants and animals you see in the hedgerows and on paths. Use apps or guidebooks (see page 134) to help you identify them. I use Seek by iNaturalist, but I know others who prefer Pl@ntNet or PictureThis.

Find mindfulness and meditation

When you're out walking it's so important to take time to look around you, clear your mind and be present in the current moment, but apps can be a very effective way of supporting this. You can use them either while you're walking or when you stop for a break to wonder at the great outdoors. See page 25 to find out more about mindfulness while walking.

APPS FOR MINDFULNESS AND MEDITATION

- **Calm** (www.calm.com): Great for sleep promotion and stress management.
- **Headspace** (www.headspace.com): Guided meditation to help with mental health and sleep.
- **Aura** (www.aurahealth.io): Packed with mindful music and meditations.
- **Buddhify** (buddhify.com). Designed for busy lives and not subscription-based.
- **Insight Timer** (insighttimer.com): Free guided meditations.
- **Portal Escape Into Nature** (portal.app): For those days when you just can't get out there or need to drift off to sleep remembering that last amazing walk.
- **Third Ear** (thirdear.com): A sound bath app. Some of the other apps do have this feature, but this one is more comprehensive.

3. Be social

If you plan to meet up and walk with others, you will be far less likely to opt out last-minute because you will want to avoid letting people down. Being part of a group also creates a 'fear of missing out' element to cancelling. You will wonder what experiences they are having and whether you will be able to keep up next time. It's a great motivator.

Join a walking group

Search for groups in your area via Google or social media. Some are targeted towards a particular cohort, such as beginners, women or specific ethnicities, so you will always find one that you can identify with.

WALKING GROUPS

I have listed a few below that have a national reach (in the UK), but these types of groups can be found around the world:

- **WALX** (walx.co.uk): National walking club and home of Nordic walking in the UK. Unisex/all ages.
- **Ramblers** (www.ramblers.org.uk): Britain's walking charity. Unisex/all ages.
- **Glamoraks®** (www.glamoraks.com): A global community of women who walk.
- **Wild Women UK** (www.instagram.com/wildwomenuk): A female hiking group in the UK.
- **Girls Who Hike** (www.facebook.com/groups/1680448035554562): A Facebook group for females only who enjoy exploring the great outdoors.

CASE STUDY: SONYA FEHR

Sonya battles with ME, but she believes being part of a walking group helps her cope and keeps her motivated.

'I joined a walking group two and a half years ago and I can honestly say it is one of the best things I have ever done for myself. Since joining I've been to places that I would otherwise not have visited and I do this with such lovely people, who share the same interests that I do. I love spending time in nature, but I just wasn't spending as much time doing this as I wanted to. Walking on your own and being mindful of your surrounds can be wonderful, but spending time with others in nature can be so uplifting.

Results, enjoyment and sociality – those are the three factors that will keep you walking, even if your schedule is temporarily derailed by, well, life. In fact, I believe you owe it to yourself to make sure you see the results, experience the enjoyment and encounter sociality, and, as I like to think I've shown you in this chapter, it's actually not that hard…

10

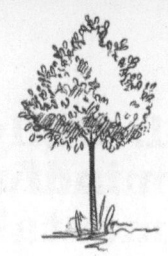

WALK THIS WAY...
For daily inspiration

In need of a reason to walk? Look no further! Daily inspirations are designed to give you plenty of great ideas! You'll find the rationale behind some of the suggestions below in the other chapters of this book and for further information on many of these activities see the Resources section. However, if you just want to get out and walk, then these will spur you on.

So that you can select an idea that suits your mood or goals each day, I have grouped them together by their main theme:

1 Daily inspirations for mindfulness and positive mental health
2 Daily inspirations to discover and learn
3 Daily inspirations to meet and help others
4 Daily inspirations to connect with the natural world
5 Daily inspirations for fitness

Daily inspirations key

To help you further I have added additional keys to indicate if the walk requires some planning or is weather dependent or seasonal:

- **S**: Seasonal
- **W**: Weather dependent
- **P**: Needs forward planning
- **L**: Laugh and be bonkers!
- **K**: Kit involved

1. Daily inspirations for mindfulness and positive mental health

Let's start with ideas for walks that are mindful and particularly good for your mental health. For more on walking for better mental health, including meditative breathing exercises and mid-walk yoga practices, go back to Chapter 2.

Make your walk a pilgrimage (P)

Connect with your forebears by making your walk a pilgrimage. While most people have heard of the famous pilgrimage walk the Camino de Santiago de Compostela in Spain, many are less aware that pilgrim routes can be found elsewhere and that all religions have some kind of destination that draws people to it for worship and contemplation.

The term 'pilgrim' is often applied to any traveller who walks in order to discover a foreign land, new way to live or spiritual enlightenment. The essence is to shed the usual trappings of daily life as you walk and ponder on a journey towards your chosen destination. Some pilgrims prefer to walk alone (although often they find meeting others en route is the most profound element of their walk), while others do so in a group. I have spoken to many who have found taking part in a pilgrimage life-changing. Research any routes near you or plan a longer walk further afield, so you can follow in the footsteps of others on a voyage of discovery.

Go on a touch safari

A great way to take your mind away from the day to day is to explore what you encounter when walking via touch, not just sight. Feel the coldness of a metal gate and reach out to touch fences and hedges. Allow your hands to brush through grasses and crops, and take time to stop and touch tree bark, noting how it varies from tree to tree. If you encounter moss, take time to sink your hands into it, feeling the delicious sponginess.

You will soon find that you are concentrating on something to touch rather than the clutter in your mind, and the sensory experience is both rewarding and calming (for more on hedgerow immersion, see page 44).

Yoga walk

Yoga and walking are a wonderful combination. This ancient mind and body practice helps improve posture, stability and mobility, as well as reducing stress and anxiety, and helping you develop mindfulness. By adding a yoga break into your walk, not only can you stretch and strengthen your muscles, but you can tap into your breath, engage with nature and enhance your holistic experience. I like including mid-walk standing postures (then you can avoid getting muddy!) after I've warmed up, such as a powerful Warrior pose followed by a calming forward fold. You can find more benefits of yoga and some postures on page 30. If you only want to add one into your next walk, it just has to be the Tree pose (of course!).

Throw away a problem (K)

Master the art of disposing of things that bother you. This walk is a great one if something is bugging you, you feel upset or you have issues that might always be there in the back of your mind. Take an eco-pen or pencil with you and walk to a lovely spot. Find a stone or leaf that appeals to you, write the issue, thought or name of the person causing the problem on it and give it back to nature. Bury it or simply leave it in the undergrowth to be taken over by nature. Listen to the satisfying splash as you throw your pebble into the sea or the rustle as leaves fly off in the wind, taking your problems with them.

Ponder as you walk

Use walking to ponder about something or just to allow your mind the freedom to wander. Many of the daily inspirations in this section work best if you learn the art of 'pondering' – a great word derived from the Latin word *pondare*, which means to weigh or weigh up. To ponder means to think about things fully, something we do not always do due to the pressure to make decisions or meet targets. Sometimes, you will come across a location that makes you want to stand and stare or stay a while, perhaps because of the view or the surrounding nature or the strong feeling it evokes, making you feel good. Make a note of these spots as places to practise pondering and treasure them.

Find the animal within (L)

Get back to basics and engage with your inner animal as a way to clear your mind. Once you reach your selected location on a walk, stop talking (if you are with somebody else) and try to clear your mind. Now imagine you are a wild animal walking along the same path. Rather than chattering or thinking about work or the shopping list, any animal will simply be using all their senses with two clear goals in mind: finding something to eat and trying not to be eaten. To do this, they will be listening to every twig that cracks, sniffing the wind to identify any other creatures or food sources, looking carefully at what is around them and being totally immersed in their surroundings. Using the methods outlined on page 41, use this walk to be more aware of your senses just as an animal would. It will keep your mind from wandering back to the human state of chaos!

Go barefoot (S, W)

Walking barefoot is one of the most profound and grounding things you can do as, of course, we were not designed to have shoes between us and the earth. So, find a suitable spot, take your shoes and socks off and give it a go! Obviously, check the ground is free from glass or other sharp objects and then take slow steps, concentrating on the sensation. Think of your feet as being as responsive to touch as your hands, as you feel the ground beneath you, exploring the coolness, wetness or softness of grass or leaves on a woodland path. In fact, your feet are one of the most sensuous parts of the body so you will soon discover the joy of exploring different surfaces like sand, moss and chipped bark.

It doesn't just feel good: research suggests this is also a great way to counteract the positive charge that comes from our phones and electrical devices throughout the day. The earth gives off a negative electron charge that is said to neutralise these – this is what is known as grounding or earthing and it is widely believed to promote better sleep, boost immunity and even improve the viscosity of our blood.

Physically, walking barefoot can improve mobility, help with conditions like plantar fasciitis, and encourage natural posture and movement. Always start gently, as your feet have been used to shoes for a very long time.

'Our bare feet are conscious of the sympathetic touch of our ancestors as we walk over this earth' – Chief Seattle, Duwamish Suquamish

Breathe with a tree (S, W)

This is a powerful way to realise how we need the sun and nature to survive while feeling a deep connection with a tree, so find a tree that you feel connected to and sit quietly at its base with your back to its trunk. Look down at its roots and as you breathe in slowly let your eyes move upwards into the canopy. Pause briefly and then exhale slowly, before bringing your eyes back towards the roots and ground. This is a powerful exercise because as you pull in the fresh air, you are taking in oxygen created by the tree as a by-product of using the energy of the sun to process the carbon dioxide in the atmosphere. This deepens the connection with the tree, and helps us realise that we need the sun and nature to survive. I find that once people have tried this, they return to the tree and repeat this often. For more on connecting with trees, see page 177.

Think with your feet

As we evolved, our feet had a far more important role than they do now – they had all the senses typically now found in our hands, and connected with our brains via touch to help us balance and stay upright. Nowadays, we do not use them fully, especially as we encase them in shoes. This exercise teaches you to reignite that connection, to 'think and feel' through your feet. While it works well when barefoot, here is a more practical version that you can practise when wearing shoes (flexible, minimal soles work best).

Imagine you have no shoes on and step forward without directly looking at the ground (pre-check the ground to ensure it is clear of trip hazards). Close your eyes, if it's safe to do so; if not, just look ahead. The aim is to ask the feet to explain the terrain below to you. Is it level or sloped? What type of surface is it: hard, soft, slippery, cold or stony? Use your other senses. Listen to your footsteps. Think about any sounds underfoot; any smells emitted with each step. Imagine what the feet would be 'feeling' without shoes.

Repeat this periodically on a walk, wherever you encounter different terrain such as grass, gravel, pine needles and mud. If you are ever on a beach, practising this on the tideline is amazing as there are a range of surfaces with distinct sounds and feel; for example, you can go from dry, soft sand onto gritty, crushed shells or small stones, through damp squishy seaweed back to wetter sand. You could walk along one surface: take a step to the side and walk back on the next surface, or walk directly through from one to the other and feel the contrast with each step. In a woodland, the path is very different under trees where pine needles may differ hugely from the leaves of deciduous trees.

When out walking, check your terrain with this concept in mind. You will soon find some great examples that you walk over regularly. Have fun and enjoy thinking with your feet.

Discover the power of slow

Harness the power of walking slowly and discover how it stimulates the brain. Consciously drop your pace for the bulk of a walk, noting how your mind wanders and you begin to process thoughts. About halfway through the walk, speed up for a short period. Notice how your focus will migrate to the physical movement and effort exerted, and your mind will be less active. Slow down again and allow your mind to be nurtured by the slow rhythmic pace.

TIP

You will find you have your best ideas when walking slowly, so leave a pad and pen out for when you return and jot them down.

Walk with a mindful app (K)

Try using a mindful app on your walks if you find your mind tries to override your efforts to focus on breathing or meditation. Many are specifically designed to be used in a static state (lying or sitting in a warm, relaxed position), so be aware that walking in a busy location or one where you need to concentrate on your surroundings could affect the experience. The Calm app has short, specific walking mindfully recordings, which are very effective. Another way to combine walking and a mindful app could be to use them when resting at your ponder spots (see page 151).

Walk with a crystal (K)

Explore the healing powers of crystals to embark on a journey towards holistic health. These natural minerals have been used for centuries to help people feel grounded and are said to balance or fine-tune energy. Ancient healers and modern practitioners believe each type of crystal has a different energy field or frequency, so can help bring harmony in specific areas. Quartz and jade are good for healing, while amethyst is said to help with negativity and grief. For those in polluted environments like cities, turquoise is said to help you detox. Some believe you are drawn to the crystals you need most, so choose and carry one that appeals to you and, as you walk, focus on the crystal and what you would like to harmonise.

Body drumming

Body drumming is a great way to relieve tension if you are feeling stressed. Try it when walking. Before leaving the house, make a fist with your dominant hand and lightly 'drum' along your opposite arm from the shoulder towards the hand, down and up one leg at a time, and gently across the torso and backside. Next, switch hands and concentrate on the opposite arm and shoulders to make sure the whole body is energised. While walking, you can drum along your arms, upper body and backside periodically, or stop somewhere relaxing and repeat the exercise.

Smilage (L)

Crack a smile in order to release feel-good endorphins. On your next walk, consciously try to smile – it will make you feel good. Even a small half smile from the corners of your mouth can have a profound effect on how you feel. It can activate the parasympathetic nervous system, which manages your body's responses, including relaxation. You will be able to use this simple tool whenever you feel uptight or stressed.

Use your gaze

Look to the horizon to reduce stress. We tend to work on screens a lot these days, or at least focus on close-up things. When we are stressed, our pupils dilate as part of the fight-or-flight process, but strangely, this can actually narrow our focus, making us less aware of what's around us.

A great way to reduce stress when walking is to actively use your eyes. Scan around you, taking time to look upwards and to the sides, using your full vision. Look into the far distance and then try to soften your focus. It also helps to stop in a safe place and close your eyes for at least a minute – this blocks out all external stimuli and helps create a feeling of calm.

Walk in the moment

Understand the meaning of being present in the moment with this mindful mantra and practice. Walk slowly, inhaling and exhaling with each step. When you are ready, take a step and say to yourself, 'I am walking into the present.' With the next step say to yourself, 'I have arrived.' Take a second to ask yourself if you truly felt in the present, with no thoughts of the past or future. If not, keep practising and, when you find that inner calm, enjoy it and acknowledge it.

Ask someone to walk shoulder to shoulder with you

Look ahead to help you and others share problems as you walk. As walking has become more recognised as something that is great for mental health, people began looking into why it seemed easier to 'open up' when walking or to communicate with certain individuals if that was something that did not come easily to them. The answer is so simple – when you walk with somebody, you are walking *alongside* them, not looking directly at them. This makes it easier to converse with people you have just met, tackle difficult subjects or simply open up about how you feel.

Those who organise group walks see this on a daily basis and marvel at the power of a sociable walk. Perhaps you know somebody who is struggling and an invitation to join you today could be just what they need. Or maybe you need to tackle something or share a problem and inviting a friend, partner or family member to join you on your walk could be a great way to start that conversation.

2. Daily inspirations to discover and learn

This section is all about discovering something you didn't know about your local area or the world in general as well as yourself. Widen your horizons, try something new and be amazed at what you can do on foot.

Walk with alpacas (P)

Allow an alpaca to take the lead for an endearing and surprising experience. I used to think this was a gimmick until I arranged some alpaca walks for a festival and saw the effect it had on people. It remained the most popular and highly reviewed walk on the schedule, and here's why. Not only are alpacas endearing, with their comical looks, curly topknots and cute noises, but they make a walk all about *them*, not you. They love to head out, but, in my experience, *they* will choose the route and will refuse to be cajoled into going elsewhere. They will also go as fast or slow as they please, and stop as and when they want to. This is a great lesson for those who love to be in control or are short of patience. After a while, the group seems to settle into a calm rhythm dictated by these wise, peaceful creatures. Let them lead and you will be rewarded for it (and hopefully avoid one of their moody spitting gestures).

Walk and wild swim (P, K)

Combine a hike with a wild swim for the ultimate experience. The benefits of wild and cold water immersion are well documented, but I think the best swims are those you have to hike to – a tiny tarn in the mountains or a cove along a craggy headland where no cars can access will reward you for the miles you have covered to get there. It also makes you appreciate the power of walking as a way to connect with places experienced only by those willing to go on foot or perhaps bike. Take a fast-drying towel, a change of clothing and a warming drink and hat if its chilly. Make sure somebody knows where you are going, that you know the waters and are a confident cold-water swimmer. Ideally, when in remote locations, swim with others that you trust.

Walk a long-distance path (P, K)

Go the distance for a life-changing experience. OK, you may not have the time to do this in one walk, but there are several amazing trails around the world, from the famous Appalachian Trail in the US to the Bicentennial National Trail in Australia (all 5330km/3300 miles of it) to be conquered. Most are easily broken down into sections, with specific guidebooks, maps and accommodation to help you plan how to conquer them. Whether that's over a few weeks, a weekend here or there or a section every year, the choice is yours, but the reward is huge either way. There is a camaraderie among those on the trails and those who provide for them as they pass.

The South West Coast Path is the longest of the UK's national trails, with over 1000km (630 miles) of glorious cliff-top walking through Somerset, Devon, Cornwall and Dorset. It features in several inspirational books, including one of my all-time favourites, *The Salt Path* by Raynor Winn. Check out all of them on the National Trails website.

Discover 'Slow Ways' (P)

Find a Slow Way near you and help it to survive. Thinking about your locality and where you are walking can be insightful if you take a while to consider the creation of the footpaths, roads and pavements that have developed over many years. While Roman roads link many cities, the smaller paths typically linked outlying farms and communities with markets and churches. Sometimes this is obvious as you stand in an open field and trace those paths, but it can take more research.

Over millennia, people have trodden paths for a reason (and for convenience) and they still do today, cutting corners across car parks or creating shortcuts. The Slow Ways organisation looks at routes used by locals both throughout history and in rapidly changing urban environments, and fights for them to be recorded and used. An army of volunteers are recording these paths in an effort to make it easier to walk more and there are now Slow Ways maps with thousands of routes to keep you walking. See if you can find one near you and help it to survive.

Try a trails and train walk (P)

Ditch the car and explore the most amazing places by taking the train to the starting point and either doing a circular route back or – far more exciting – walking to a station further along the line. You can pick your location for a good day hike and then search for routes on local walking sites or see the designated walks on Railwalks. Linked to Slow Ways, this network of routes has been added by volunteers and is a great way to discover an area while making use of public transport. Routes include nine miles into the centre of Bath, a section of the South West Coast Path in Devon, and walks in the Highlands and Wales.

Walk like a dog (L)

When creating these daily inspirations, I hope that I can inspire people to be as excited by their daily walks as dogs are. Perhaps not waiting by the door, lead in mouth, but anticipating the joy and freedom of stepping out and discovering so much.

Watch dogs to see how they sniff the air to immediately find out who is about and then sniff at ground level to track any creature who may have passed that way. They combine all their senses, watching, smelling and listening (or not listening when it suits them). They also display a joy at their freedom in the great outdoors, meeting other dogs, running, playing, rolling and tumbling.

While I'm not expecting you to pee up bushes or chase a ball, try to anticipate what you might discover today and use all your senses as you look at the world around you. Be thankful for this chance to be free and take the opportunity to engage with others en route.

Compose a poem

Walking is quite rhythmical and it allows the mind to be creative, so why not attempt to think up a poem? It can be about something you see when out or what you are feeling, but it's rewarding and often surprising what you can come up with. By playing around with and repeating words, you are clearing your mind of everything else too.

Don't get hung up on the technicality of poetry. Your poem doesn't even need to rhyme (although that's a great place to start). We are not talking the complex structure of a sonnet and who cares if it's only a limerick? Give it a go and see how time flies as you think of a line and then add a rhyme (see what I did there?).

Walk to a pub (P)

Do I really need to add this as a daily inspiration? It's possibly one of the most enjoyed weekend walking pastimes. However, that means it is often a habit featuring the same walks and the same couple of favourite pubs. So, do a bit of research and seek out local circular routes that start and finish at a pub or pass one en route. There are books on this very subject, and these stops can make a walk very special in both summer and winter. You could even go one step further and plan a route with a pub tour, where you stop off at a couple, or plot walks in locations away from home. Pubs usually have good car parks, and provide refreshments and facilities too.

Walk a food tour (P)

Build a walk around refreshment stops for multiple benefits. I got this idea when I organised a festival in Seville and we were taken on a walking tapas tour. A lovely evening walk was broken up with stops at stunning hostelries where we were served a plate of local tapas before moving on.

You could pre-plan your food tour and phone ahead, or make it more ad hoc depending on where you are walking, but it's a great way to get to know somewhere you may be visiting and support local businesses.

A longer day walk could involve two to three stops for coffee and/or breakfast, lunch and even supper at the end.

Walk a maze (P)

Walking in a traditional hedge maze is disorientating and puzzling, which is exactly what they were intended to be. Many were planted as part of formal gardens on large estates to provide a challenge for guests who would walk into the labyrinth and try to find a way out of paths that suddenly end or turn back on themselves. The maze at Cliveden in Oxfordshire was made of 1000 yew trees, 2m (6ft 7in) high, creating 500m (546yds) of winding paths, so it is a great way to get your steps in while using your puzzle-solving skills.

Mazes made of tall plants, like sunflowers and maize, and annual ones are more popular these days, providing a sensory experience. Some mazes are made through wild-flower meadows, created from cut turf or even a mix of dense woodland and tunnels, like the one at Cragside in Northumberland.

For a more mindful maze experience, you can walk to an ancient turf maze called the Breamore Mizmaze near Cranborne Chase in Dorset, which it is believed was cut by medieval friars from an Augustinian priory. Although you can't walk on it, you can trace the winding curves with your eyes as you take a rest from the stunning route to its location. Mazes can be new too, like the dry-stone wall maze being built by a team of volunteers at Dalby Forest in Yorkshire.

Walk and listen

Learn or escape as you walk. I am not a fan of wearing headphones as I like that connection with nature and feel safer when I am using all my senses, but I appreciate that others may find that time walking can be combined with learning, listening to music or catching up on favourite podcasts. If you are going to do this, make sure you are visible to others and maybe combine the walk with a positive podcast about healthy living, being active or connecting with nature. I know one walker who times his evening stroll with his daily dose of *The Archers* on Radio 4 and I love the fact that it adds value to his walk.

Learn a language

The rhythmic action of walking is known to help with creativity and learning, so why not use your daily walk to brush up on a language? You could listen to an app or use prompt cards. Take time to name things that you pass or even stop every now and then to look them up. Of course, the best way for a language to sink in is to speak it out loud and what better way to practise than when walking in the middle of nowhere?

Ancient trails (P, K)

Step back in time with each step forward. Some trails have additional historic merit, so there is daily inspiration to be gained by planning a walk on one. Hadrian's Wall and Offa's Dyke in the UK, for instance, are ancient boundaries or barriers between warring tribes or nations. Their elevated positions and ancient stamp on the landscape make them beautiful, atmospheric and steeped in historical interest. Like other long-distance paths, they come with maps, guides and ideas for short sections to be covered via circular walks too.

Lesser-known ancient trails are located all over the UK and many combine road sections with footpaths. The Harrow way (or Harroway, which means old road) is said to be the oldest road in Britain, dating back to 600BC and is linked to pilgrimages and possibly Stonehenge. Some sections today form major A roads, while other are still walkable and full of history, including parts of the South Downs Way.

Across America, there are trails that detail history as gold diggers and immigrants sought new lands to explore, while in Australia, many of the highways are based on songlines which are trails made by Indigenous Australians, who are said to have used stars and stories to navigate them. Book an outback experience walk with local experts to really feel the landscape. If you want to really expand on this concept, consider a walking trip to cover the Great Wall of China or similar. There are walking holiday companies that can lead you or support you en route.

Walk a holloway (P)

In the UK you can find ancient paths that are so well trodden they sit deep into the landscape with steep banks either side and overhanging hedges or trees. Known as holloways, these are magical tunnel-like paths where the base is often wider than the gap of canopy above, and they are well worth seeking out. Their name comes from the Anglo-Saxon *hola weg*, which means a sunken lane, and they are stunningly beautiful as well as atmospheric due to the shady mossy undergrowth. You feel cocooned and immediately realise that your footsteps are simply scuffing the surface of footprints past.

I live in Dorset in the UK, so I am lucky to be in an area that hosts over 65km (40 miles) of them, including the famous Hell and Shutes lanes, said to have been carved out by the travails of both quarrymen and smugglers. Natural England is mapping them all in a bid to ensure they are never destroyed.

Walk with the classics

Always wanted to read a classic or enjoy a book with no interruptions? Now you can. Use one walk a week to catch up on an audiobook that you might otherwise find too time-consuming to read. Of course, you could always enjoy one of the inspirational walking books I feature in my book list, too (see page 214).

Walk on ley lines (P)

Enjoy the experience of walking a ley line and only try to understand them if you need to. I spent some time in the modern city of Milton Keynes and was fascinated to find out that when positioning their new boulevards the architects were inspired by ancient monuments like Stonehenge and Avebury. Were they hippies at heart, like me, and following 'ley lines'?

I have always felt some kind of energy from the earth in certain places and explored both the spiritual ideology with more factual theories written about how many ancient sites were often linked by straight lines (a theory first written about by Alfred Watkins in the 1920s, when the term 'ley lines' was coined). Whether man-made via ancient tracks or pilgrim routes, forged by water (see Walk to find water on page 168) or magnetic energy, there are several distinctive 'lines' that can be discovered and walked.

You can research ley lines local to you or start at an ancient monument and check out routes leading to other features on the map, such as churches and other ancient sites. Suffice it to say that our ancestors trod those paths for a reason, be it something practical like trade or something more spiritual.

Take a history tour (P)

Take advantage of local experts by booking yourself on to a walking tour. Most areas have them and there is always more to any area than you might think. Whether it's ancient artefacts, Tudor buildings or an industrial heritage, a history walk helps you understand a place so you can imagine those who trod the same paths in days gone by.

If modern history is more your thing, you can enjoy themed walks based on bands like the Beatles, or TV shows like *Peaky Blinders* (2013–22) and, more recently, *This Town* (2024). The 2Tone trail in Coventry is a must. One town also has a walk dedicated to the pop star Harry Styles, so I rest my case when I say there is a reason for everyone to walk.

Go on a night walk (K)

Walking at night changes your perspective. The lack of light heightens your other senses and the world around you behaves differently. Chirpy birdsong subsides and the owls begin to hoot as foxes and badgers start to emerge. In urban areas, traffic noise and general bustle calm down too. Wearing a head torch is essential where the paths underfoot are tricky or you need to be seen by others, but if you are somewhere safe and tranquil it is lovely to switch it off and allow your eyes to acclimatise to the dark for a while. Obviously, safety is paramount, so walk with others and wear hi viz if there is any risk for you. See also Walk with a full moon on page 189.

Stargaze on a dark sky walk (P)

Explore the universe as you walk under a dark sky. A walk that will stay with me forever is when an astrophysicist stepped in after somebody asked what the particularly bright star we could see was. None of the group knew what he did for a living, but suddenly the world around us came to life. His knowledge of the stars, universe, galaxies and milky ways astounded us all. Now, I seek out places with dark sky designations, where there is no light pollution and you can see much more than a few stars. It is truly inspiring – even if you have no idea what you are seeing.

There are over 160,000 square kilometres of protected land with night skies in 22 countries on six continents. From cities that manage their urban lighting sensitively to designated parks, dark sanctuaries and reserves – to find them use the Dark Sky Place finder website. You will also be able to find walks led by dark sky experts often with the chance to visit observatories.

Codiwomple – discover walking words (L)

Amuse yourself by musing over walking words. My favourite word is *codiwomple* – an old English term for walking with purpose to an unknown destination. It sums up this book, which aims to add purpose to every walk, but leads to who knows what!

A great way to ponder this word and others is to think about how you are walking today and use some of the many 'walking words' that have made it into dictionaries over the years. You might start out strolling, ambling, sauntering, dawdling or moseying, but end up traipsing or trudging as the going gets tougher. Just try not to waddle or mince as that's not good for posture. Each of these conjures up a different way to walk, so maybe try a few on your walk today.

> **TIP**
>
> Why not practise your walking style by taking a promenade in your finery – a popular pastime in Victorian times, which is still practised in some countries (see Enjoy a passeggiata on the next page)?

Walk instead of... (P)

Save the planet and gain fitness with every step by choosing to walk. This daily inspiration is based on the concept of active travel, which will ideally become part of your walking week. Where possible, consider a journey that you usually take by car, tram, bus or train and replace at least a section of it on foot. One of the best tips I used to give my weight loss walking groups in an urban town was to get off the bus two stops early. Check out Sustrans, which has lots of ideas for swapping carbon-guzzling modes of transport for the healthier, more sustainable and original mode: walking.

Walk with your inner child (L)

Jump in puddles, crack ice or zigzag along the path in an unorthodox way. Children show joy when outdoors and find pleasure in the simple things. Today, try to avoid the cracks in the pavement or break into a skip when nobody is looking. Maybe attempt some hopscotch or another childhood game. Even walking like certain animals can combine fitness and fun; in fact, there are fitness programmes based on animal movements. It might seem like pure madness, but we replicate these things in some of our fun fitness sessions and the laughter it generates probably does more good than the exercise. So, the message is: do something that incorporates the free spirit of a child and generate some of those uninhibited giggles that will leave you feeling brilliant.

Enjoy a passeggiata (L)

Go continental and enjoy the Italian tradition of a passeggiata. This is a leisurely stroll, usually in the evening, with the purpose of socialising, and supper and aperitifs can feature. Once experienced, never forgotten, this way of walking displays all the elements of social connection, and the fact people seemingly dress for the occasion likens it to the displays other animals put on. In more reserved countries you may need to be sure your smiles and greetings are not met with horror, but try to embrace the theory of socialising when walking.

Climb a 'mountain' (K)

Top a hill for elation and reward. There's nothing like the elation of getting to the peak of a hill or mountain. Setting yourself a challenge is a great motivator and achieving your goals will boost your confidence. However, it's important to always select something that, while tough for you, is not beyond your capabilities or you could end up feeling negative. Start with local hills and travel further afield once you know you have the stamina to climb for longer. Be aware of how things can change as you go above certain heights. For tips on hill climbing see page 55.

Go on a fossil walk (K)

Finding or viewing something that is circa 130 million years old is one of those moments that will always stay with you. As somebody lucky enough to reside on the Jurassic Coast, I can wholeheartedly recommend a walk with a geologist or fossil expert. I now never see the ground below me or hills or cliffs without picturing them millions of years ago as the glaciers shaped and folded them, leaving fossils of sea creatures discoverable inland. A walk I lead regularly provides an opportunity to literally follow the footprints of dinosaurs. Fossils and geological features are not just found in coastal areas, so check out what is in your area and be inspired. Abide by the rules, though, and do not collect or create damage.

Walk and paddle (P)

Enjoy a walk to a waterside spot where you can hop on a paddleboard or canoe. Some centres allow you to drop it further along a lake shore or river and walk back, which is a great way to see the landscape from different perspectives.

For longer treks, planning to cross a body of water via a paddle craft can provide a great route plan. There are specific walk and paddle events as well as groups. Between the difficult times of Covid-19 and the January 2021 attack on the US Capitol, US senator Tim Kaine did an epic walk, cycle and paddle across Virginia, the state he represents. He made the journey in sections and describes it in his book, *Walk, Ride, Paddle: A Life Outside*. Be inspired by Kaine and plan a journey on foot and water traversing an area that may be difficult or tedious on foot alone.

Embrace walking songs (L)

On your next walk, amuse yourself with thinking about how many songs mention walking. Sing them out loud, hum them to yourself or just try and name as many as you can. I will start you off with some of the most obvious, but the fact there are so many proves that walking is a fundamental part of living and features in all aspects of our lives.

The best walking song ever, in my opinion, has to be 'I'm Gonna Be (500 miles)' by the Proclaimers, but here are a few others:

- 'Walking on Broken Glass' by Annie Lennox
- 'Walk On By' by Dionne Warwick
- 'These Boots Were Made For Walking' by Nancy Sinatra
- 'Walk Like an Egyptian' by the Bangles
- 'Walking on Sunshine' by Katrina and the Waves
- 'You'll Never Walk Alone' by Gerry and the Pacemakers
- 'Walk On the Wild Side' by Lou Reed
- 'Walk All Over You' by AC/DC

Walk and fly (K, W)

Be at one with the wind for both mental and physical benefits – another daily inspiration where initially you might think I've lost the plot, but hear me out. Walking to the top of an open windy place and flying a kite is another of those childhood memories that should be revived on occasion. Why is it so joyous? Because as you work with the wind you are at one with the elements.

Kite flying also improves eye function for those used to focusing on tiny screens. Tracking the kite in the sky relaxes eye muscles and helps with eye strain, while you are also working on coordination, posture and upper-body engagement. You must stand firmly on the ground, so it can be grounding too.

TIP

No need to lug a massive heavy kite up to the hilltop: tiny pocket-sized kites are available in stores that embrace nature, such as the National Trust or RSPB.

Walk to find water (K)

Try the dowsing for water as you walk. Water dowsing is an ancient tradition, which is also used by modern water boards today. There are lots of 'explanations' about why, if you walk with metal dowsing rods held out in front of you, they will cross as you walk over a water source, but no scientific proof that it works or does not work. Some believe we subconsciously move them because we have read other subtle signs around us or are picking up on something like electromagnetism. Others believe that we have simply developed to be able to locate water and when we focus on doing so with rods, it works. I have tried it and seen it work with others, so take the view that we don't need to always know why. Dowsing rods can be easily sourced and are light too, so why not give it a try?

Walk and scream (K, S)

If you enjoy being scared, why not take a walk with some ghosts? Whether you decide to dress up for Halloween, join a guided trick-or-treat-style walk or opt for a ghost hunt, there are plenty of ways to enjoy a 'spooky walk'. In most cities, you can find an organised scary historical walk, such as the Jack the Ripper trails in London, which take you along dimly lit alleyways in areas not usually frequented by visitors. Other cities also have their favourite tales, which cover everything from highwaymen to plagues and executions. The City of York claims to have the oldest haunted walk in the UK, Edinburgh excels with its witches tour and Bristol offers 'walks with the dead'.

Walk in their footsteps (P)

This daily inspiration is almost mindful, because it makes you appreciate that you are just another person to tread a trail. I guarantee that every established path has some history, funny story or 'smilage factor' attached to it. Was it a route to market, built by the Romans, used by smugglers, drovers or highwaymen, or was it involved in the war? Just one example near my home revealed an old bridge where drovers were charged a copper to cross and soldiers marched to the civil war. Let your mind wander, make up stories or do some research to bring the route to life. Stimulating minds and memories is a vital element in the fight against dementia, so it's great to exercise your imagination as you feel more connected to where you are.

Browse a market (P)

Get your steps in as you browse a market – far better than a trolley dash around a supermarket. Whether you want to get up early to experience the City of London waking up at the famous Smithfield Market or plan a walk that takes you to a local farm shop or farmers' market, there's something brilliant and grounding about a potter and a chance to learn about products. Markets provide an insight into local traditions, culinary treats and interesting artisan products. Antique markets can provide endless hours on foot and a workout as you carry your purchases. There are specific tours of the most famous markets too.

Go on an artistic walk (P)

Release your inner artist or feast your eyes as you walk. If you can't make it to Paris to walk around the artists' easels at the Sacré Cœur and along the Seine, why not check out art festivals where you can walk from gallery to gallery, viewing works by local artists. Or perhaps street art is more your thing? There are tours in many cities that take you past the best graffiti sites, including Banksy tours in Bristol and London.

Maybe you could join an art group who walk to locations worth painting or pack a plein-air easel and take yourself off for a mindful experience. In Worksop near Nottingham, you can take a walk from a modern gallery to a cave with ancient art on the walls. In Dorset you can find a sculpture park with walks that take you past majestic artworks.

3. Daily inspirations to meet and help others

Walking is one of the best ways to engage with other people and to make a difference to both your life and theirs. It is a calm activity that requires no kit and it's something most of us can understand, too. Enjoying it with others can also help the environment, encourage somebody to talk about their problems, become a challenge or simply be a lot of fun.

Participate in a silent disco walk (K, L)

A great way to get together with others to enjoy music and exercise is to attend – or even arrange – a silent disco walk. It's a fun way to socialise, have fun and get fit in a group as you share the sounds with each other, but not everyone around you. Obviously, there is some technology involved – generally wireless headphones and a receiver – one person is usually in charge of the playlist. If this idea has struck a chord but you walk on your own, you can also join sessions with DJs worldwide via other apps.

Walk to find treasure (P, K)

Geocaching is a great way to incentivise yourself or others to go out for a walk and be part of a worldwide community. It is basically an outdoor treasure-hunting game where followers stash and locate hidden waterproof boxes in wild locations. According to the Geocaching Association of Great Britain, there are over 3 million geocaches hidden worldwide and more than 5 million people who play the game.

Enthusiasts put small items of interest with nominal value in boxes, hide them and post their locations on a website or app using coordinates. Others find them, take the items and put something back in of a similar value, while taking time to complete the log and make a comment. Obviously, you need a smartphone and a signal to play this, but the boxes are in some stunning locations on the best walking routes, so there are two incentives to get out. Another bonus is that geocaching can help boost your navigation skills, so it's great for family walks.

Become a walking volunteer (P)

As somebody who organises group walks and festivals, I know the power of passionate volunteers – we have hosts and walk leaders who want to spread the word about how powerful and life-changing walking can be.

One way to promote walking to youngsters is to set up or get involved in a 'walking bus'. Typically, this is a crocodile line of schoolchildren walking to school with an adult 'driver' and volunteers keeping them in line as they stop off at various points to collect children and deliver them to school. It's not just a case of a few parents getting together or a social media post, though; these groups need insurance, safeguarding, vetting and an adult-to-child ratio of circa one to four, depending on age.

Lots of charities, care homes and organisations organise fundraising walks such as memory walks (see opposite), which are often in need of volunteers. Or you could become a heritage guide and lead history walks or tours. The possibilities are endless. Check out your local council for a host of volunteering options and guidance or visit Sustrans or the NCVO volunteering directory.

Take part in a charity walk or distance challenge (P)

Signing up for a challenge walk is a great way to commit to walking more. It will not only provide a goal to work towards, but it will also encourage you to introduce the three elements of fitness and longer walks into your weekly regime.

Most large charities hold challenge walks both in the UK and abroad, which are in amazing locations with plenty of support from marshals and others. They are a great way to meet people and make lifelong friendships as you cover the terrain and interact at the start and finish locations. T-shirts and medals are added bonuses and, of course, the chance to raise money for the miles you cover is always a positive. Action Challenge is the company that organises many of these, so check out their Ultra Challenge Series or see Macmillan's Mighty Hikes, which raise money for people living with cancer.

Go 'netwalking' (P)

If you work in an office or on an industrial park, why not inspire your colleagues to hold netwalking meetings or set up a group with other local businesses to do a lunchtime circuit? By walking and talking you can forge links while you take a break from the office and improve your fitness. Even if you work from home, you can reach out to other homeworkers, and bring exercise and connection into what can be deskbound, lonely days. Even those who are not in the work environment, like retirees or stay-at-home parents, can benefit from walking with like-minded people, so get networking and arrange your netwalking meetings.

Try synchro walking (P, L)

You ideally need somebody else for this one – preferably four or more to really feel it. Over the years, I have noticed how walkers often fall into step with each other, not just stride patterns, but sometimes left and right legs too. Marching soldiers are trained to synchronise every movement and while it can look stiff and formal, our brains sometimes enjoy this rhythm.

Since 1996 team precision walking has grown into a pastime and many universities have teams that perform moves as intricate as a marching band at the Trooping the Colour. In Japan, where they call it *Shuudan Koudou*, synchronised walking is massively popular. It's a fantastic and fun way to perfect teamwork and precision, and is mesmerising to watch and demanding to participate in – one team even covered 1200km (750 miles) during practice. Just walking in step is a good start, but if you fancy it, you can plan some exercises too.

Join a memory walk (P)

In Chapter 4 we covered the science behind brisk walking warding off dementia – a positive way to not only remind yourself why you need to step it up on occasion, but also how walking is an effective way to boost memory and interact with those suffering from this debilitating condition.

Memory walks are mass charity walks organised across the UK by Alzheimer's Society, where people walk for and with relatives with dementia. It is quite moving. There are also lots of groups who also organise regular local memory walks and I have seen first-hand how positive they are for those with the condition and their loved ones. The international equivalent is known as the Walk to End Alzheimer's.

Walk and celebrate (S, L)

Festivals and carnivals all over the world involve processions and joining one can be a great way to feel part of a celebration on foot. Whether you go carol singing in your local community, rattle a collection tin as you follow the floats making their way through town, or simply stroll through the Diwali lights, walking is the best way to feel part of the action.

Go further afield and you could be pelted by tomatoes in La Tomatina, a festival in Buñol in Spain and the biggest food fight in the world. At the end of spring, Holi festivals are held all over the world and involve a procession where people cover each other with brightly coloured paint. See also Walk a wassail (page 182) to appreciate how walking-based celebrations have always been part of life.

Litter pick walk (K, P)

Litter-picking volunteers cover miles every week in their local areas as they gather rubbish discarded by others. The action of picking up litter requires bending and reaching, too, so it boosts fitness and mobility while helping to clean up the environment and help nature, but above all, litter-pickers tell me it's a sociable activity. Whether it's meeting up on a beach, walking the roadside verges or clearing the local country park, armies of litter-pickers meet up and improve outdoor spaces. It's a rewarding way to get your daily steps in.

4. Daily inspirations to connect with the natural world

As there are so many daily inspirations that relate to nature and the senses, I have broken them down into four categories:

a Making a difference to nature
b Finding a sense of awe
c Connecting with the seasons
d Connecting to your senses

Making a difference to nature

Add some value to the steps you take by joining the fight to protect, record or learn about endangered species.

WALK WITH BUTTERFLIES (S, P)

What better way to make a walk worthwhile than by signing up to spot butterflies? Some butterflies only feed on certain plants; others fly at certain altitudes. Noting those you see and exploring what has attracted them will enhance your joy at watching them flutter past and give you a deeper understanding of their habitats. The rare and endangered ones are so special, and there are ways to record and report on your sightings to help protect them. Every year, an army of volunteers regularly walk specific areas to officially record the butterfly population. Butterfly Conservation is a UK charity with leaflets to help you identify the butterflies you see, as well as ways to record them.

WALK AND RECORD (P)

If you love wildlife and want to make a difference, you could become a nature recorder or citizen scientist! Naturalists have been recording species of plants, insects and birds for centuries. This has helped us take action to protect habitats when we see potential decline. These days there are lots of opportunities for less-experienced amateurs to help with data collection and it's a valuable way to enjoy a walk. Most local wildlife organisations have regular schemes you can link up with and I have seen recorders lucky enough to watch puffins, whales, eagles and dolphins for hours.

The aim is to simply record three main facts about a species (which you obviously need to be able to identify). After giving your name, the date and the species you are recording, all you need to make a note of is where it is, using the grid reference or what3words link. Different organisations have different ways to collect data and will often hold recorder training days. Globally the data is shared and you can find out more at the Global Biodiversity Information Facility. There are apps and sites such as iRecord, which is a UK national records website scheme in which you can record every type of wildlife. You can build your own list of records and a map showing them, which others can see, enabling them to help wildlife and those who manage it.

FEED THE BIRDS (K)

Whether it's ducks on a pond, urban pigeons or wild birds in a hedgerow, taking time to feed the birds provides a welcome mid-walk break. If using birdseed, make sure you are not wantonly planting something inappropriate in a certain habitat, but typically it's fine to scatter native wild birdseed somewhere it will hopefully remain dry long enough for the birds to find it. Many field margins are planted specifically to provide seed for birds, and pollen for bees and other pollinators. Check out what's there so you know what you can put on your wild bird menu.

SEED BOMBING (K, P, L)

Throwing a few seed bombs as you walk is a great way to release your inner child and boost diversity. You can buy these in eco shops and garden centres or make your own (great recipes are available online). Make sure the seeds are right for the area you are bombing. I use hollyhocks and valerian around dry walls and urban waste spaces, and poppies, cornflowers and knapweed in field margins and hedgerows. There's nothing like spotting one of your 'babies' when you walk the route later in the year.

Seed bomb recipe

You can make seed bombs with flour or recycled papier-mâché – most wildlife trusts or eco organisations will have a recipe. I think clay works best and, if possible, clay that is local to where you are 'bombing'. You can get powdered clay in most garden centres too.

Using coffee grounds adds some fertiliser for the seeds, but you can skip this and just use peat-free composts and clay to bind it.

Ingredients

2 parts good peat-free compost
4 parts clay or clay powder

If using coffee grounds add 1 part – if not increase the compost to 3 parts

Method

- In a large tub mix all the ingredients up well, adding water to bind, particularly if the clay is dry.
- Next add 1 – 2 parts of local wild flower seeds (never any invasive species).

- Roll into balls and lay out on card or paper to dry – egg boxes are great for this.
- Leave to dry away from direct light for 24–48 hours.
- Wrap in waxed paper and pop in your backpack or foraging pouch (see page 134). I use mesh bags from supermarket fruit and veg aisles to store batches, too.

Finding a sense of awe

We have all experienced that moment when a view or encounter with a creature takes your breath away. Seek out the power that nature has to amaze yet ground you.

WALK WITH ANCIENT TREES (P)

Search out an ancient tree for a grounding experience. Trees dating back thousands of years are a sight to behold and it's worth a walk just to be in their company. While yew trees in Scotland and Wales are said by legend to be up to 9000 years old, the oldest recorded trees can be found all over the world, from Chile and China to Iran. Some are in secret locations, but others – such as the largest tree in the world, the General Sherman, a giant sequoia in the Giant Forest of Sequoia National Park said to be 2000–3000 years old or the rare Wollemi and Huon pines in Australia – are protected, but available to view.

Many of the ancient trees in the UK are on land that was once private, but is now open to the public and managed by organisations like the National Trust, which has helped to protect them. Whether it's the famous Old Man of Calke, which sits on the site of Calke Abbey in Derbyshire, or the Major Oak in Sherwood Forest, which is linked to the legend of Robin Hood, I love to watch the reaction of others as they encounter these specimens and urge you to search for one near you. You can find a list of them by UK county, along with walks that include them, on the Ancient Tree Forum website. The Woodland Trust also has an inventory of ancient trees. Most countries will have records and there are many articles online that direct you to the oldest trees near you. If you're based in the US, check out the organisation American Forests, or if you're in Australia, have a look at the monumental trees website.

Ancient trees are not only found in rural locations. Hampstead Heath in London boasts an ancient tree trail that takes in several specimens and provides information on each one.

WALK BY WATER (P)

Today try to locate some water to walk beside. Many studies show that being by water improves our well-being, with those living near the sea scoring higher in relation to health and happiness. People are more likely to feel like being active by water and its presence can be cooling on a hot day. If you are lucky enough to be by the sea, you can benefit from clearer air and calming waves, but inland waterways have other benefits such as providing natural navigation. Canal paths are well maintained, not hilly (obviously) and take you into tranquil countryside or historic urban areas. Check out organisations that are responsible for their upkeep like the Canal & River Trust in the UK for great walks by water. In the US, you can search for canals state by state on the American Canal Society website and the Inland Waterways International website is useful, too.

EMBRACE THE RAIN (W)

Select a rainy day and embrace the smell that emanates from the ground around you, especially if it has been dry recently and you are near porous surfaces like stone or concrete. The lovely fresh, earthy smell released, called petrichor, was first identified by Australian scientists in the 1960s and has health benefits. It's created by a mix of plant oils and tiny microorganisms call actinobacteria that release a chemical compound called geosmin, which is distributed as if by mini aerosols as each raindrop hits the ground and creates a splatter. Humans are particularly sensitive to this smell and it takes us back to that instinctive connection to nature. Studies also show that serotonin levels are increased by geosmin, which could be because it ionises the air, adding a negative charge to air molecules. So, never let rain put you off – pop on those wellies and take time to enjoy the smell and mood boost it will give you.

GO ON A FUNGI FORAY (S)

Uncover a whole new world under the autumn leaves as you discover fungi. Best in autumn when they really start to show off with both edible and deadly toadstools and other shapes, these amazing life forms, essential to our landscape, are working underground all year round. Each visible fungi is supported by a network of mycelium (like roots) which feed both them and the plants and trees around them via a symbiotic and wonderful relationship (it's fascinating, but far too complex to outline in full here). Go out and marvel at the visible fungi and imagine that network underground, improving soil, providing food and water and sending signals to other life forms. Use an app or book to learn about mushrooms, but do not pick or eat them – they are far more useful where they are.

TRY A NATURAL FIRST-AID WALK (K)

Take time to think about familiarising yourself with natural ways to ease aches and pains, build awareness of how to treat incidents when walking and think about what to take with you. I have a range of small natural sprays and tinctures to help with cuts, blisters, bruises and bites. It is beneficial to carry products containing lavender, aloe or calendula for skin conditions, arnica for bruising, and camomile teabags in case you need to deal with shock.

Plantain grows in pavement cracks, fields and gardens *everywhere*, and can be used to make a multi-purpose skin salve that is great for skin abrasions, bites and stings. There are two types to be found: broadleaf or greater plantain *(Plantago major)* or narrowleaf or ribwort plantain *(Plantago lanceolata)* – look them up on a plant app. Pick up this wonder plant when out walking and take it home to dry and make into an oil. There are plenty of recipes available online, but this is my favourite. If you get stung when out, chew a leaf and apply the salve (make sure you are 100 per cent sure you have the right plant, though).

Plantain oil recipe

1. Collect about 30–50 plantain leaves from either variety.
2. Wash them gently and leave them to dry.
3. Tear them into pieces and press them into a glass bowl or jar and put the bowl into a saucepan. Fill the saucepan with water up to the top of the jar, but not so high it can get in to the mixture. Alternatively, use the bain marie method as if you're melting chocolate (I prefer this as it's gentler on the compounds in the herb and cleaner, too).
4. Heat gently for about an hour, making sure you top up the water up in the pan and stirring occasionally. The leaves should lose their bright green colour.
5. Remove from the heat and sieve to remove the leaves, which you can discard, and obtain the oil.
6. Wipe the glass bowl clean, pour in the sieved oil and add about 20g beeswax pellets or grated up old beeswax candles. Pop the bowl back into the saucepan and stir to melt together.
7. For a nice fragrance and added skin care benefits, you can add a few drops of pure lavender oil.
8. Have clean jars or small tins ready as you need to pour the mix in quickly before it sets. I use tiny jam jars for home and little salve tins for backpack use.

DISCOVER A FORMAL GARDEN (P)

Get your steps in while immersing yourself in the wonder of a formal garden. Experience how humans have learned to work with nature to create stunning canvases that have changed in fashion over the years. In the UK many National Trust or English Heritage properties have gardens and landscapes guaranteed to tire you out, but there are magnificent famous gardens all over the world, including the Alhambra in Spain and Monet's Garden in France. Many formal gardens have visitor centres and some have walking trails and wilder spaces, as well as stunning borders. In the UK there is also a National Garden Scheme, where people open their gardens for charity – maybe you could combine a couple of local gardens in one route? Many now have wilder areas to encourage biodiversity and it's good to compare how you feel in each area.

WALK ON THE WILD SIDE (P)

Discover rewilding locations where nature has been allowed to take back control. One of my walkers gave me a book about rewilding many years ago with a comment like, 'This is just so you.' I was immediately hooked and transformed my own garden, while watching the concept take hold and change the way people manage land, verges and gardens.

These days, there are great examples that can be visited and enjoyed, with walks and safaris that not only allow you to enjoy the wildness, but also help you learn how to bring elements into any green space you may have access to. The Knepp estate in West Sussex, a pioneering example of a farm that has been completely transformed, is now a centre for education and is open to the public, while Highlands Rewilding has now transformed three large estates in Scotland and offers retreats. The RSPB was determined to transform hill farms in the Lake District to encourage the return of golden eagles and the story of the rewilding of Haweswater is outlined in the book, *Wild Fell*. You can now visit and support these projects by taking a wild walk.

WALK IN STORMY WEATHER (W, K)

Watch wild waves crashing on shore or trees bowing in the wind for an exhilarating experience – as long as you are not too close. While I would not advocate chasing a thunderstorm or walking directly under lightning, there is something invigorating about embracing bad weather. If you dress correctly and understand the safety factors, it can be grounding to experience how powerful nature is. If you are caught in an electrical storm, make sure you know what to do to keep safe (see page 140).

WALK WITH A CAMERA (K)

Capture the beauty of nature on a photography walk. Because walking specifically to take photographs creates a link between you and the world around you, it is the one time I embrace phones or cameras. Because you want to capture the landscape, flowers, insects and sky above, you look at it with creativity and mindfulness. Taking time to capture the shot is calming and takes your mind away from other stresses in life.

Try to go on specific photography walks rather than snapping everything you see on every walk, which devalues both the walk and the experience. If you take images to share when out walking, always ask yourself why you are doing it and whether it is taking you out of the moment. If they often contain you as well as the nature you are enjoying, ask yourself how much value it has to others. The only time I embrace having humans in photos is when nature provides a perfect picture frame – the heart-shaped walkway mentioned on page 195 or a hole in a gnarly tree trunk, for instance.

Connecting with the seasons

In a world where we can eat tropical fruit in mid-winter, it is easy to lose contact with the seasons. In this section the walks are designed to help you focus on the glory of the season you are enjoying. This is how our ancestors lived and it's good to eat, live and walk seasonally!

ENJOY A WINTER WONDERLAND (S)

Make the most of those sparkling winter frosts when cobwebs and seed heads sparkle with ice crystals in the low winter sun. Those magical days tend to tempt even the least active away from the fireside, as frost not only looks wonderful, but there is something delightful about crunching across grass and cracking open the frozen puddles. It evokes memories of childhood and is one of many ways to connect with the outside world in the colder months. While it is important to not restrict your excursions to such days, because they are often few and far between, it is a *must* to make the most of them.

Winter can be dark, grey and wet, so when the ground is white and the sky blue it can give you a boost of vitamin D and lift your mood. The structure of bare trees looks spectacular and furrowed fields take on a different perspective when tinged with white, as if dusted by icing sugar. Things sound and smell different in winter, too, so take time to breathe in deeply through your nose and out through your mouth to get that essence of nature shaking off the abundance of summer and preparing for regrowth. Stand and listen to the wind, which is no longer hindered by leaves on the trees as it whistles through the valleys.

WALK A WASSAIL (P, S, L)

Celebrate the heritage of cidermaking and enjoy an ancient tradition by joining in a wassail. Many acts of procession and celebration link us to the seasons and nature. There are too many to include in this book, but one that stands out to me as brightening up the winter and helping us to look forward is the wassail. In the UK, this involves walking with lit torches and chanting an ode to the apple trees before feeding them some of the current batch of cider. It sounds bonkers, but similar ancient traditions can be found the world over and they really do connect you to the seasons and local produce.

ENJOY THE DAWN CHORUS (P,S)

Step out early and immerse yourself in birdsong. In spring, the birds start singing at dawn, usually peaking at about 6.30 a.m., when it's time to start feeding. As migrants arrive from overseas, the chorus increases as resident males let incomers know it's their patch and they all try to attract females. Singing loudly signals they are in good shape and ready to mate.

At dawn, when the air is typically still, it can be mesmerising to hear the birdsong, which is well worth the early start. The chorus is different in woodlands, open country or wetlands due to the different species residing there, so there are multiple chances to get up early, pick a spot and sit with a flask as you let the sound wash over you. Check out the RSPB for walks led by knowledgeable guides.

SKETCH A TREE THROUGH THE SEASONS (K, S)

Connect with a tree four times a year as you watch it change through the seasons to create a sense of calm and gain a better understanding of nature. Identify a tree that stands out in the landscape with shape and presence. There is no need to be a Picasso, just sketch what you see each season. It's a great way to immerse yourself in that calming cycle of nature that you will learn to feel part of. Whenever you start, the tree will present differently: boughs heavy with shimmering leaves in summer, crispy colours in autumn, a wonderful skeleton in winter and emerging buds in spring. Learn to rejoice in those changes and notice how they make you feel.

ENJOY A CORDIAL WALK (S, W)

A not-to-be-missed summer experience that engages your sense of smell and enjoyment of the seasons has to be an elderflower walk. Take a stroll where these flowers are in bloom and pick a few to make a wonderful cordial or tea. Elderflowers drip from the tree in a scented haze of tiny star-like flowers that smell creamy and sweet. They can turn musty, so sniff before you pick. Avoid picking elderflowers on windy days when the pollen will be blown away and the fragrance and taste reduced. Pop them in a bag and use them immediately. Do not wash – just shake to de-bug.

How to make elderflower cordial

Ingredients

Fresh elderflower blooms (enough to fill a 1 litre (34fl oz) jug)
- Lemon juice (half a lemon to every 500 ml/17fl oz of cordial)
- Lemon zest (to taste)
- 350g (12oz) sugar

Water (enough to cover the elderflowers in the pan)

Method

1 Pick the elderflower blooms, shake to de-bug and lightly pack into a 1 litre (34fl oz) jug.
2 Remove the stems up to the point the main stem meets the smaller ones that attach to the flowers.
3 Pop the flowers into a large pan and cover them with water, adding lemon zest to taste.
4 Simmer for 30 minutes, topping up with water, if necessary, to make sure the flowers remain covered.
5 Strain the elderflowers through a tea towel. Squeeze to get as much juice out as possible.
6 Measure to see how much juice you have and add the sugar and lemon.
7 Gently simmer this mix to dissolve the sugars.
8 Remove any scum that forms on the surface and leave to cool.
9 Pour into sterilised bottles, leaving about 1cm (½in) at the top to allow the cordial to breathe.
10 Seal with a cork or screw top. The cordial will keep in the fridge for up to three weeks.

GO ON A BERRY-PICKING WALK (S)

Become a hunter-gatherer for a rewarding walk that will make your tastebuds zing. Is there anyone who has not plucked a ripe blackberry from a bush? They are so abundant that any autumn walk will provide an opportunity to do so, whether urban or rural. Ardent jam-makers will go out armed with big gloves and return ladened with bowls or bags full, but I like to just graze as I walk and remind myself it's a seasonal bounty. Blackberries make an excellent tea too. Sloes, which are found on blackthorn bushes, are famous for their ability to turn gin into a warming dark red liquor. Just steep them for at least six months with some sugar added to sweeten.

FOLLOW THE CELTIC TREE CALENDAR WHILE YOU WALK (S, P)

Take time to research, learn and discover more about trees – once you start you will never look back. Discover more about their physical strength and uses, how they support each other (and other species) and the ancient spiritual connections they hold. A great way to feel connected to the phases of the moon and ancient folklore is to embrace the Celtic tree calendar, which links the moon phases with trees.

This is based on the UK seasons, but you can research and modify this calendar based on your location. Alternatively, look into ancient calendars and links to trees such as the calendars created by indigenous people that deeply connect humans with other creatures, plants and nature. For instance, the Ancestral Tree of Life carving called the Izapa Stela 5 stone preserves a historic record of the Maya Five World Ages and calendar systems. It is also said to illustrate the story of humanity and its origin in the early Americas. CSIRO, Australia's science agency, is also a good source of information on Indigenous Australian seasonal calendars.

The Celtic tree calendar has 13 phases, starting on Christmas Eve. Each is linked to a type of tree or plant, the sacred powers it was said to have and the attributes that were then applied to those born within its 'phase'. You can find calendars outlining these and various texts and meanings to research further, but I think it's nice to just know the phases and to check in with the different trees or plants during their 'season'. It's also lovely to know which one relates to you and to find one to visit on your walks.

You could schedule a walk where you find an example of each of the 13 trees or plants or where, at the start of each phase, you seek out that particular one. Groups can celebrate those born in that phase and so on. Of course, you can enjoy them on any date and experience their phases throughout the year, too. Below, I list the most common depictions of the tree moons for you to use and I hope you visit them all via these 13 phases:

1. BIRCH WALK: 24 DECEMBER-20 JANUARY

The Celtic tree calendar starts at a time when the winter solstice has passed in the northern hemisphere and it's time to look forward to more light. The birch is a tree that symbolises protection and rebirth (it is always the first to regrow after a fire, for instance). The pale stems are magical and well worth seeking out on a dismal day.

2. ROWAN WALK: 21 JANUARY-17 FEBRUARY

Rowan trees are magical, whether you believe they are associated with Brigid the Celtic goddess of hearth and home or not. Their hardy nature means they can be found clinging to hillsides with unusual foliage and bright berries. They are linked with travel, personal power and protection, so walk to find one and check out the personality it exudes, wherever it may be located.

3. ASH WALK: 18 FEBRUARY-17 MARCH

These magnificent trees have been under threat recently from ash dieback, so it's even more important to locate and watch over those near you. Sacred and magical to many, and said to be what Odin's sword was made of (in Norse mythology), they are also linked to toolmaking (including magic wands). Given the chance they can live for over 400 years and because their leaves allow light through and fall early, they are often surrounded by other plants on the forest floor. Enjoy their straight, strong trunks and look up through their delicate leaves. Pop back in late summer to see bunches of 'keys' hanging off them, too.

4. ALDER WALK: 18 MARCH-14 APRIL

Linked with the spring equinox, this tree flourishes on riverbanks where its roots are in water. The wood is therefore great for boat building and even forms the base of the City of Venice. Its often-swampy habitat meant it was also linked with fairies and it was sometimes feared because when cut the wood turns orange as if it is bleeding. Alders are often found in stunning locations, where the sound of water adds to the feeling of durability and strength they impart. Older trees sometimes lean over the water, even forming natural bridges.

5. WILLOW WALK: 15 APRIL–12 MAY

Willows love wet soil, and in the Northern hemisphere its often pretty wet during the old Celtic willow moon phase. Willows can be cut back hard and will regrow quickly, so are traditionally linked with healing and growth. From the majestic weeping variety used for cricket bats to the often-coppiced goat and osier willows used for making baskets, our relationship with willows is strong. There's nothing quite like sitting under a weeping willow, almost hidden under a wonderful fringed canopy, to ponder.

6. HAWTHORN WALK: 13 MAY–19 JUNE

Traditionally linked to Beltane (May Day) and the start of summer (halfway between the spring equinox and the summer solstice), this tree bears scented flowers that fill the air with vanilla and are delicious in tea too (see page 46). May Day traditions saw maidens dancing around hawthorn trees before maypoles took over and folklore links the thorny tree to male potency. It was said to be unlucky to cut and bring indoors, and some farmers will leave one in a field rather than cut it. I don't think you can beat sitting on a gnarled trunk of a hawthorn to hear the insects buzz in the flowers! Hawthorn is easily coppiced, so forms hedgerows that can be found pretty much anywhere.

7. OAK WALK: 10 JUNE–7 JULY

Trees are now in full bloom and the oak often stands above the others, leading to its centuries-old links with kings and rulers. In myth and legend, it is linked to gods like Jupiter and Zeus, who were also said to control lightning. In fact, oaks are often struck by lightning due to their height, yet many survive for centuries and are a wonder to behold. In all cultures, oaks symbolise strength, protection and success – I recall my gran telling me to carry an acorn in my pocket for good luck in exams or interviews. Like many, I am captivated by the shape of majestic oaks and love to connect with them.

8. HOLLY WALK: 8 JULY–4 AUGUST

Very much associated with winter and Christmas, this prickly evergreen gem was thought to be a reminder about the immortality of nature, because it stayed green as others began to colour. The wood was used for weapons and lucky charms, and sprigs were displayed in the home as protection against witches. Found everywhere in varying sizes, it is a more difficult tree to embrace but a joy to behold nonetheless. The shine of the deep green waxy leaves and the way the trees often form interesting shapes make them worth seeking out. The wood is also great for making walking sticks.

9. HAZEL WALK: 5 AUGUST–1 SEPTEMBER

Another hedgerow staple, often coppiced to create straight stems used to make hurdles and thatching spurs for roofs, the hazel also produces delicious nuts. The nuts, which appear before many other fruits and foods, were said to be good for warding off rheumatism, but I never seem to get to them before the squirrels! Linked with wisdom and knowledge, hazel stems or rods were used for water divining (see page 169) and also said to symbolise fertility in medieval times. They are happy, unfussy trees with stories to tell and I love spotting the straight new growth among old gnarly trunks.

10. VINE WALK: 2–29 SEPTEMBER

Not really a tree, but linked to a time of harvest and connected to the autumn equinox or Mabon, when fruitfulness and food are important, grapevines or hop vines symbolise strong emotions, such as happiness and rage. Vine leaves were traditionally used to promote ambition or set goals and feel more balanced at a time when there were equal hours of darkness and light. Try to locate a vineyard or hop garden and enjoy the fruitfulness (and maybe a glass or two, in honour of the vines).

11. IVY WALK: 30 SEPTEMBER–27 OCTOBER

Again, technically not a tree, but an important plant that is much maligned, ivy is fascinating and easy to find. Take a walk and look at how ivy scrambles up its host, with suckers on its stems. Evergreen like holly, it was used to decorate homes and ward off spirits, but its clinginess was also linked with love, friendship and romance, so enjoy a walk where you befriend ivy and understand its value.

The Woodland Trust say ivy does not harm the trees, but, of course, it can limit light and take some nutrients. However, it also produces nectar and fruits when very little else is around, and so supports bees and birds in tougher times. I was once walking with a group who stopped to marvel at bees around tiny green and yellow flowers and on another occasion were fascinated by birds feeding voraciously on purple and black berries. Both incidents took place on ivy, which would normally be passed by without a second look, and the walkers had no idea they were ivy flowers or berries.

12. REED WALK: 28 OCTOBER-23 NOVEMBER

Reed was typically used for thatching, valued for its protective qualities. Traditional reed instruments were used at wakes and the haunting sounds have linked reed with the cycle of life in many traditions. Still used today for wind instruments, it is found by water and is magical to watch as the wind blows through it.

13. ELDER WALK: 24 NOVEMBER-23 DECEMBER

Elder is another common plant found in hedgerows and gardens, often sown by birds or animals who have eaten the berries. Prized for its fragrant flowers (see Enjoy a cordial walk, page 183) and power-backed fruits, it is a favourite of foragers. Traditionally it was said that having an elder near your home would ward off the devil, but I prefer to think of it as the colourful tree. The bark, leaves and fruits are the source of the natural earthy colours found in traditional Harris tweed. The elder moon association is probably due to its ability to renew when cut at the same time as the winter solstice, meaning there will be more light and regrowth.

WALK WITH A FULL MOON (S, P)

Check out the full moons that appear every month. In fact, there are sometimes two to enjoy. To help you understand their significance to our ancestors and nature, I have explored the name of each full moon below to make it even more magical to walk beneath. Just like the trees, most cultures will have a name for these moons; some are also known as supermoons due to their size, colour or brightness. Most of the more common names used today originated from terms used by native Americans, but I have also added some of the common Celtic and Anglo-Saxon names.

It's easy to find out when a full moon is likely to appear each month via apps or internet searches and, once you know what they are called, you can walk out and imagine those who named them while staring up at the same thing as you are. Think about whether any of the names seem more relevant to you and where or how you live.

JANUARY: THE WOLF MOON

It is thought this moon was linked to the fact wolves were heard howling in the depths of winter when snow was on the ground. It is also referred to as the 'stay-at-home moon', probably for the same two reasons. As you walk under this moon, think how lovely it is to return home to warmth and comfort, and how much easier most of our lives are today.

FEBRUARY: THE SNOW MOON

Once again linked to the weather conditions and harshness of the season, this moon is also known as the storm moon or hunger moon. Because it comes before the spring equinox, it was referred to as the Lenten moon too (although some link this name to the March moon). Under this moon it is good to think that change is coming soon.

MARCH: THE WORM OR PLOUGH MOON

The name of this moon signifies the slight changes appearing as conditions improve and the fact it was the final moon of the winter. Perhaps worms started to appear once the snow melted, and people began working and ploughing the land again. Other names are the sap moon, the Paschal moon and the last moon of winter. Take some deep breaths and enjoy the fact that under your feet things are beginning to stir.

APRIL: THE PINK OR BUDDING MOON

The various names for this moon relate to the fact that new growth is clearly visible and the earth is springing to life. Flowers begin to appear, so some cultures named it the pink moon as their landscape turned that colour due to specific buds opening. The various names all refer to seed, buds and growth, apart from some tribes in coastal areas, who called it the fish moon. Breathe in the positivity of nature and thank it for continuing its circle as you promise yourself you will enjoy the new shoots on your next daylight walk.

MAY: THE FLOWER MOON

May is when nature is in full swing and a late evening walk when the hawthorn is in bloom will show you why this moon was named. Some cultures called it the corn planting moon; others the egg or milk moon. Walking under this moon will reward you with the scent of flowers. Seek out a hawthorn hedge if they grow locally or aim to walk by flowering plants for the full experience.

JUNE: THE STRAWBERRY MOON

Strawberry-picking season reaches its peak during this time and the name signifies early fruitfulness. Roses also bloom and in some cultures it is called the rose moon. Another name is the dyad moon. Take a punnet of strawberries out with you and delight in the sweet early summer, ideally near a rose garden – bliss!

JULY: THE BUCK OR HAY MOON

These names reference the cutting of hay and the velvety down growing on the antlers of buck deer at this time of year. Another name is the mead moon, presumably after the ancient honey liqueur – perhaps take some with you to enjoy a taste of summer as you smell the freshly mown hay?

AUGUST: THE STURGEON, RED OR GRAIN MOON

This moon has many names, from the grain moon and red moon (possibly due to the summer hazes) to the sturgeon moon (this large fish was readily available in the American Great Lakes in August, so the name is thought to relate to that). As you walk, think about how nature is providing on both land and sea.

SEPTEMBER: THE HARVEST MOON

The good light of the harvest moon allowed farmers to harvest their crops late into the night. However, the harvest moon does not always occur in September as the name tends to be associated with the full moon closest to the autumn equinox. This falls during October once or twice every 10 years. Sometimes, the September full moon was called the corn moon, wine moon or song moon too. As you walk under this moon, think about how nature provides so much of our food and how we could be working in partnership with it more.

OCTOBER: THE HUNTER'S MOON

As mentioned above, some years the harvest moon (also named the bold moon) falls in October instead of September. Once the harvest was in, attention turned to filling the larders before winter, which meant animals that had grown large during summer were hunted. Now it's time to be grateful for how easy it is for us to gain good food and not have to panic-store. Enjoy this often bright moon and perhaps resolve to eat more seasonal foods.

NOVEMBER: THE DARKEST OR BEAVER MOON

Don't be put off by the name; it's good to go out and embrace any full moon, even if things are colder and dimmer. Also known as the mourning moon or beaver moon in areas where beaver fur was prized for warmth, the focus is clearly shifting towards the winter to come and how times may be tougher. As you walk under this moon, use it to reflect on how lucky we are today in that seasons don't affect us as much as they used to, although we could be more careful with the light and heat we enjoy.

DECEMBER: THE COLD MOON

Embracing the full moon at this time of year is more rewarding than you might think. Winter now takes a firm hold and temperatures plummet. This moon is also called the long night moon, because it spends more time above the horizon, opposite a low sun, as we approach the winter solstice. The full moon name often used by Christian settlers is the moon before yule. Why not plan a solstice walk (see page 186) and celebrate the fact that the nights will soon be shorter.

BONUS WALK: WITH A BLUE MOON

Some years there's an extra moon to enjoy and this walk is not to be missed. The moon takes circa 29.5 days to orbit Earth, which typically gives us the 12 lunar months we know. However, the lunar month is slightly shorter than the month in a solar year (the measurement between the summer and winter solstices is approximately 365 days, 5 hours, 48 minutes and 45 seconds), so every two to three years we can enjoy an extra full moon. These do not have names, so are referred to as blue moons, and they should be embraced and enjoyed via a blue moon walk!

Connecting to your senses

By truly engaging the senses – sight, sound, smell, touch and taste (see page 46) – we can transport ourselves from the day to day and feel more immersed in nature.

BRUSH THROUGH LAVENDER FIELDS (SMELL) (P, S)

For an unforgettable sensory experience, walk through lavender fields. OK, getting to Provence in France at the time the lavender fields are in bloom is not always feasible, although it should be on your bucket list. However, there are lavender farms elsewhere these days and there is nothing quite like the experience of walking along rows of this pungent health-giving herb and tapping into the sense of smell. The fragrance is heady, yet known to be calming and sleep-inducing, while the colours are vibrant and varied. Gently brush past the blooms, inhaling deeply and allowing your eyes to focus closely on the flowers to one side before pulling your gaze away to include the wider rows around you. The sensory experience is unforgettable, and often you can reward yourself with lavender-infused treats and oils from the farm shop too.

ENJOY A CLOUD-GAZING WALK (SIGHT) (L)

Take time to look at the clouds when out walking. Identify shapes or patterns that remind you of things and let your imagination run – it's mindful. Notice how often clouds form the natural shapes we explored in Chapter 3; some resemble skeletons or fish scales (the mackerel sky) and I have seen trees, flowers and even a perfect shell. My best formation looked like a pod of dolphins leaping over waves and I once saw a perfect cross that was not formed by aircraft vapour trails. Take time to remember the formations and look them up so you learn more about what they mean. For those who love tech, the Cloud Appreciation Society has an app where you can share cloud forms and use AI to find out more about over 50 types.

WALK WITH MINIBEASTS AND BUDS
(SIGHT) (K)

Pop a mini magnifier in your pocket (sometimes called loupes or jewellery magnifiers, see page 134) and engage with minibeasts. These tiny eyeglasses will help you to see the world you are walking through in a totally different light. Stop and look deeply into the plants or pathways. You will discover a fascinating array of creatures going about their business or plants in different life phases that are less visible to the naked eye, with petals unfurling or pods bursting with seeds. You can see the tiny hairs on a plant stem and even the pollen on the bees' knees!

This childlike activity stimulates your senses, slows you down and connects you with nature. Trust me, once you have experienced the tiny 'forest' you see when you look closely at moss, you will never set off without your magnifier again. If you want to get into identifying some of the wonders you see, there are guides available from the Field Studies Council.

CONJURE UP TREE AND HEDGE SHAPES
(SIGHT)

Look closely at the trees and hedges, using your imagination to spot shapes as you wander. Looking closely at the shapes that nature creates will open up a wonderful world. Left to grow, trees and bushes burgeon, but they are often shaped by the elements and other creatures, like the oak tree in a field of grazing animals where the base of the canopy is dead straight at nibble height, while the rest of it is freeform. Hawthorns on windy hillsides bend away from the wind and create amazing shapes that can often look like other things as you approach them or see them silhouetted in the skyline.

I have some favourites that never fail to surprise when I point them out to others. The two stags complete with magnificent antlers formed out of a couple of straggly trees and a windswept T-rex dinosaur, who leans over the roadside with his head, front legs and tail shaped by the wind (oddly enough, close to where you can walk on dinosaur footprints). Other favourites are where trees meet over footpaths to create a framed view of the path ahead – one I walk through regularly forms a perfect heart shape and never fails to make me smile.

WALK UNDER BLOSSOMS (SIGHT/SMELL) (S)

Enjoy the Japanese tradition of celebrating the blossom. Once the blossoms start to appear, search out your nearest cherry trees or apple orchards. One blossoming tree is a wonder to behold on a walk, especially if you stand beneath it and look into the tiny festoons of flowers, but if you are lucky enough to source an orchard or avenue it's almost intoxicating.

In Japan, cherry trees are revered and festivals take place throughout the country, starting in the south and following the blossoms as they open. Called *Hanami*, this tradition goes back centuries and culminates in family picnics under the blooms. These days there are similar festivals in many towns and cities worldwide, including New York, but my best cherry blossom walk was in a churchyard in west London.

WILD TEA PARTY WALKS (TASTE) (K, S)

A great way to use your sense of taste when out walking is to enjoy wild teas. During spring, the hedgerows explode with colour, fragrance and birdsong, and you can use all your senses by looking deep into the hedge, listening to the birds and smelling the flowers, taking time to enjoy nature's bounty. Here I explore the variety that are available during spring, summer and autumn. Read more about hedgerows teas on page 46.

SPRING

- **Hawthorn:** These bushes will also give you a heady smell to enjoy. Pick a sprig or two of fresh flowerheads, ideally with some unopened buds (you can include a couple of leaves too) and simply add to your tea flask (see page 131) or take home for a relaxing seasonal brew.
- **Nettles or dandelion leaves:** These are full of health and vitality. Use them in the same way as hawthorn.

- **Gorse:** This is also in flower, so, taking care to use gloves, pick the flowers for a coconutty tea (best brewed via a teabag rather than dropped in a cup).

SUMMER

- **Linden tea:** *Tilleul*, as the French call it, is my favourite relaxing brew. Look for lime trees, which are often in avenues and older parks. You will smell a sweet honey-like fragrance and see tiny yellow flowers, loved by bees for their sticky pollen. Pick a few with the first two leaves and some unopened buds to infuse. They are lovely fresh, but the flavour intensifies if you dry them too.
- **Pine or spruce teas:** As the vivid green tips of new growth appear on spruce trees, pick a few off and infuse for 10–20 minutes for a tea that is full of vitamins C and A. Make sure you know your species, as the yew is toxic and can look similar. Never pick too many, as the tree needs to grow. You can collect pine needles to dry as tea, too.
- **Meadowsweet flowers:** These also make a delicious, sweet vanilla-like tea during summer.
- **Pineapple weed:** This relative of camomile sprouts in gateways, pavement cracks and driveways. Look it up, as it does taste like pineapple.

AUTUMN

- **Heather:** Heather tea can be made from the flowers and young leaves – fresh or dried. It is a delicious and pretty tea that mixes well with other flowers such as gorse, which tends to grow in similar areas, making it a proper moorland tea.
- **Hops:** These need to be picked before they start browning. The flavour is in the 'cone' under the papery petals, which imparts all the flavour and properties that make it widely used in sleep-inducing tea blends.
- **Rosehips:** These provide a real boost of vitamin C. It is something we drank in the past in a syrup form, but is not great fresh due to itchy hairs in the middle. Chop them up and dry them before adding to brews in a teabag. You can buy eco-friendly, compostable teabags or infusers online.

5. Daily inspirations for fitness

The following daily inspirations will specifically boost your fitness.

BAG A MUNRO OR WALK A WAINWRIGHT (P)

If you venture to Scotland, a great way to walk for fitness is to walk a Munro – this is the name for peaks over 910m (3000ft) in height. It has become a pastime to 'bag' as many as you can and as there are 282 of them there is ample opportunity to build up towards the highest: Ben Nevis.

Similarly, in the Lake District, Alfred Wainwright detailed 214 fell-top walks, which are now legendary walking routes. His original guidebooks are quaint and followed by purists, while others use apps to combine the walks in order to get more than one done in a day. Either way, these challenges add motivation and make walking a passion for many. Similar trail bagging can be found all over the world, so you will never be short of a reason to head out and up.

JOIN A WALKING SPORTS TEAM (P)

Take your walking to another level by joining a walking sports team. If you find adding twists, turns or bursts of speed via the exercises and fitness walking sequences in this book difficult to master, taking part in a team game that includes them could help. Most sports, from football and netball to rugby and hockey, now have teams who play at walking pace. Trust me, the slower pace does not spoil the enjoyment or effectiveness of the activity and you will certainly know you have taken part.

USE POLES (K)

I make no secret that my go-to exercise solution is to use fitness poles. Think of a cross-trainer in the gym and imagine that you can work 90 per cent of your muscles at the same time, while also feeling lighter on your feet and breathing fresh air. Using poles well is a game-changer, so take a minute to read about them in Chapter 4.

GO RUCKING (K)

Quite a trend these days, rucking is all about walking with a weighted vest. It can really boost your CV workout, but will only add strength benefits to the legs, although that's great if you are pulling a few squats or lunges en route. A word of warning: you can feel quite sweaty. Don't be fooled by expensive kit; you can achieve similar benefits by carrying your kit and a few bands in a well-fitted rucksack. That way you can stop and work the upper body too.

Note: You may also see ankle weights promoted for walkers. My advice is to steer clear as they impact on good walking posture and can cause strain or injury. Likewise, walking with handheld weights can cause wrist, arm and shoulder injuries. It is far better to walk naturally and stop to incorporate effective strength work (see page 85) into a walk.

TRY STEP AEROBICS

No, not on a plastic step in a stuffy aerobics studio – my outdoor step aerobics concept involves using any flight of steps you might encounter en route. Not only will you get a cardiovascular boost, you will be able to work on core and leg strength too. Find the fitness walking sequences on page 94 and soon you will never miss an opportunity to add a few exercises to your daily walk.

TRY SPEED WALKING

Picking up the pace to add a cardiovascular boost to a walk is highly effective. There are different types of speed walking, so make sure you understand how to master speed effectively. Typically, 15-minute miles are classed as speed walking and you need to practise this and build up to avoid injury. Olympic race-walking style looks quite odd and is based on always having a full foot on the ground to avoid being classed as running. To that end, it is a learned technique and involves quite a bit of 'wiggling'. Power walking, on the other hand, is based around using the arms more to increase pace and I often see it performed badly, resulting in pumping arms and less-effective leg action (see page 15). Speed is a powerful fitness tool, but it is best used in bursts (see page 54).

CONQUER SPEED HIKING

Like the other forms of fast walking mentioned, speed hiking is something to participate in if you love speed and are motivated by moving at pace. As the name suggests, it is based more around the wilder trails and is essentially the walking version of trail running. On established trails, speed hikers have been recording the fastest times for years and some hikers also participate in fast or speed packing, which involves travelling as light as possible.

It's a great way to work out and see a lot of country in the shortest space of time, and is growing in popularity as an activity in some areas. Just like the speedier walking modes, there is a higher risk of injury, especially if going fast on uneven ground, so build up slowly and make sure you consider safety precautions before setting out.

ENJOY HILLWALKING (P)

Whether you are new to walking or a seasoned hiker, hills will add a huge amount of extra effort to any walk. It is a great way to boost fitness at any level and will reward you with breathtaking views too. You can use hills as a workout tool – walk to the hill, climb it and descend, for example – but you can also take up hillwalking as a pastime.

On page 55, I outline the best ways to tackle hills (both up and down) and there are some workout exercises that use slopes to add intensity. My advice is to learn to love hills, because they always add something to a walk, so head for the hills and give it a go!

BE STILE-ISH (L)

Don't shy away from stiles. They can add both interest and intensity to a walk, so seek out routes that feature them. A good walk in the country is bound to encounter a stile or two; I view these as an additional workout challenge as many involve a good step up and a high leg lift. In fact, an experienced instructor I have known for many years created a whole workshop based on types of stiles and how to conquer them. A walk I do regularly is peppered with 13 stiles of different heights, and the post-walk aches are certainly in different places.

WALK BACKWARDS

Try facing the wrong way and walking backwards. Not the whole walk perhaps, but throw in some sections where you walk backwards to challenge your muscles in a totally different way and add a workout element to any walk. See page 22 to find out more and get it right.

TRY BALANCED WALKING

If you don't have the time or inclination to include the fitness walking sequences on your walk, at least stop and do a static balance exercise or two. Your body will thank you for it.

Simply walking along a white line, placing one foot directly in front of the other while maintaining good posture and taking normal steps will work wonders. Spice it up by placing the heel of the stepping foot close to the toes of the foot on the ground and keep repeating so the feet are close together. It's best to keep your hands out to the sides when doing this. If you want to add a further degree of difficulty, try doing four steps forward and four steps backwards on the line to challenge your balance in different directions. See more on balance on page 63 and fitness walking sequences that challenge balance on page 94.

Hopefully I have managed to inspire you to turn your walks into experiences and given you a way to unwind or boost your fitness. Be ready – inspiration can strike at any moment. Almost every day I discover another reason to walk and if there's anything I've missed, do let me know and we can continue to walk this way together.

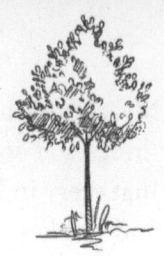

APPENDIX
Total body
walking plan

Total body walking is a way of using your daily steps to improve your mind, your body and the environment around you. If you're keen to take your walking – and the benefits it can offer – seriously, then you may wish to create a total body walking plan to help you stay motivated and on track.

In essence, a plan is a structured approach to help you build walking into your daily life. It also ensures you adopt a holistic approach to walking as it encourages you to include all elements of fitness, mindfulness, and the connection with nature that walking has to offer. To gain full benefits I would advise a plan should try to include the following four components:

1 Walking at different paces to boost your cardiovascular system (see page 53).
2 Strength exercises to build lean, toned muscles and boost metabolism (see page 61).
3 Balance exercises and range of movement exercises to keep you mobile (see page 91)
4 Something for your mental health – this could be specific mindfulness practices, yoga poses or simply things that give you joy or make you laugh (see Chapter 2).

My approach has always been to empower and inspire people to do things, so I don't want to be too prescriptive. I also know from experience that every individual starts with a different level of fitness, different likes and dislikes, and different goals, which could vary from 'I want to start walking again after illness' to 'I am training for the Camino de Santiago pilgrimage route.'

I never intended this book to be a traditional exercise book, because I feel fitness can be achieved by simply being more active, considering your own needs and getting outside more – with a few total body walking plan tweaks! However, I appreciate it might help if I answer some frequently asked questions and provide some example plans to help you get started with creating one for yourself.

FAQs

Q. Do I need to walk every day and if so for how long?

A. We were designed to be on our feet and to move every day, but fitness levels and your lifestyle will be factors in deciding whether you can go for a walk every day. You may have heard messages about aiming for 10,000 steps a day, but that can take up to 1 hour 40 minutes for an average walker and circa 1 hour 10 minutes for a fast walker. As 2000 steps a day have been proven to lower the risk of premature death from cancer and coronary heart disease, even a short walk can be beneficial. It's perfectly fine not to walk every day if you can't fit it in.

Q. How long should a plan last?

A. It takes around 21 days to start forming a habit and feeling comfortable with a new regime and about four to six weeks to really see clear physical benefits (mental ones are immediate!). I would recommend planning a weekly programme based on the days you can commit to a walk and aim to repeat that for at least four weeks. Try to add progression every week – via speed, duration or intensity such as hills (see page 55).

Q. Does it matter if I lapse for a week or so?

A. All that matters is that you don't stop walking. If life gets in the way, do not beat yourself up for not following a plan. If you can, try to at least get out for a walk – things will fall into perspective and you will feel more positive and more likely to follow the plan again. Think of walking as your mood-boosting motivator and remember that one positive steps leads to another.

Your goal

As your plan will be personal to you, the first thing you need to do is consider what you want to achieve. Most people I work with simply want to be more active and want to feel good about themselves, but others do have a specific goal, such as 'I want to lose weight by next year' or 'I am doing a charity hike and I need to train for it.' Some might have a specific medical condition to consider (see Chapter 7), so may have goals related to that.

Spending time exploring your personal goals is important, because it will help you build a plan that will deliver the specific results you are looking for. So, grab your notebook and be honest with yourself.

Write down the answers to the following questions:

- How will having a plan help me? (This should relate to your overriding goal.)
- How many days a week could I include a walk of 30 minutes or more?
- Do I have a specific end date for my goal?

Your answers will help you to shape your plan and, to highlight this, here are examples of three people with different goals and how their personal plans were shaped as a result.

JENNY'S PLAN

Jenny wants to lose weight. She doesn't have time to go to the gym, but currently walks her dog twice a day for at least 30 minutes and longer at weekends.

Jenny is advised to adjust her pace on some of her walks and include some pace exercises. The dog will also love that. Although there are hills in Jenny's area, she avoids them, but if she includes a hill at least once a week it will give her that cardio boost.

She has ruled out using poles, because her dog needs to be on the lead quite a bit and she doesn't want to use a waist harness. She often throws a ball for the dog. When she picks the ball up, she could perform a few squats and lunges, and there are likely to be benches on her walk that she can use for a few press-ups. This will add variety into her walks, too.

The bonus with dog-walking is interaction with your best friend and often other dog walkers, which is great for mental health. It can be easy, though, not to notice the nature around you, especially if you are in a hurry, so Jenny is reminded to slow down sometimes and enjoy the moment.

RESULT: The addition of strength exercise to build lean tissue, tone and speed up metabolism, plus an increase in cardiovascular components, turns Jenny's dog walk into effective exercise.

JIM'S PLAN

Following illness, Jim, a former runner, wants to get the buzz he got from running again, but knows he needs to take things slowly.

Jim is advised to take fewer longer walks and walk a little five days a week. As that becomes easier, he can build the distance up on three walks a week and used the other two to work on his fitness and strength, keeping them fairly short, but adding in exercises.

After six weeks he was ready to push himself further with pace exercises and sequences. He introduced poles and now uses them on every walk because he feels the same energy rush and mood benefits as he got from running. He still stops to do some strength exercises twice a week and does not shy away from the hills or steps.

RESULT: Jim is able to build his fitness back just as effectively, but with a regime that is kinder to his body than running.

JO'S PLAN

Jo hates exercise, but knows she has to do something about her health and fitness. She sits at a desk all day and slumps on the sofa at night. Menopause is affecting her mood and waistline, and she feels she has lost her confidence, too.

Jo is advised to simply go for a walk whenever she can fit it in around family and work, and not to measure anything except how she feels after the walk. As her mood lifts she will probably begin to look forward to getting out and having that time to herself. She will also feel she is doing something for herself if she embraces the mindful breathing exercises and yoga poses.

Time is of the essence for Jo, so she probably can't increase the time she walks and after a couple of months the initial weight loss may begin to slow down. If that happens, she could try adding poles along with pace and strength exercises to her walks (if she tries these at the outset, she probably wouldn't have the confidence to try them). Joining a walking group may also help her experience exercise as something pleasurable.

RESULT: Improving her mood by simply getting outside is the first step in giving Jo the motivation to tackle her fitness and weight goals. Not being stressed at the outset makes her more likely to keep on walking.

Your plan template

Now it's over to you. Here is an easy-to-remember weekly plan for somebody new to walking. This plan works on a six-days-a-week basis over four weeks with set days used to focus on certain elements. Each week there is progression to encourage results without adding too much time or distance to the walks. You could use names like Mindful Monday or Workout Wednesday to help you remember what your focus is each day.

> **TIP**
>
> Build in warm-up and cool-down stretches, and ideally complete Chapter 1 before you start the plan.

If you're new to creating a plan, you can just use the template that follows or you can adapt it to fit your particular goals. If you can't yet manage walking for the shorter time indicated each day, do what you can and build it up, but if you can do more than the longer time indicated, go for it – it's *your* total body walking plan!

WEEK 1

Day		Walk duration and pace(s)	Key element/Focus
Day 1	It's the start of your walking week – be kind to yourself and take the time to walk slowly and plan the week ahead	20–45 mins Depending on fitness level **Postural pace**	**Balance/Flexibility** Concentrate on posture exercises and thinking about what you can see and hear around you
Day 2	Add some strength and toning exercise to boost metabolism and work the upper body	20–50 mins Depending on fitness level **Postural pace**	**Strength** Add some strength exercises like a basic squat and a basic press against a tree
Day 3	Increase the heartrate, burn calories and boost brain health	15–30 mins Depending on fitness level **Purposeful pace**	**CV** Stop mid-walk and add a CV exercise like step aerobics or a hill climb
Day 4	Strengthen those large muscles to increase calories consumed	20–50 mins Depending on fitness level **Postural pace**	**Strength** Add some lunges (10 reps) and bench dips (10 reps) mid-walk
Day 5	Mix it up with something to affect your mood and reward yourself!	30–60 mins Depending on fitness level **Postural pace**	**CV** Try to include a hill or some steps during the walk and try something new from the daily inspirations (see Chapter 10)
Day 6	Rest or long walk day	60 plus mins **Postural pace**	Enjoy a long but leisurely walk taking time to engage with nature
Day 7	Rest or long walk day depending on what you did on day 6	As above if it's your walk day	As above if it's your walk day

Assuming you have two days together where you have more time, if you have two rest or long walk days and they are spread across the week, simply choose which is rest and which is long walk.

CHECK IN WITH YOURSELF

At the end of week 1 ask yourself the following questions:

1 Does walking with good posture and balance feel more natural?
2 Am I more aware of my posture?
3 Has my sleep improved?
4 Have my energy levels improved?

If you answer yes to 3 or 4 you are doing really well. If you only answer yes to 1 and 2 refer back to the practices.

WEEK 2

Day		Walk duration and pace(s)	Key element/Focus
Day 1	It's the start of your walking week – be kind to yourself and take the time to walk slowly and plan the week ahead	25–50 mins Depending on fitness level **Postural pace**	**Balance/Flexibility** Concentrate on posture exercises and thinking about what you can see and hear around you Add a static balance sequence (see page 93) mid-walk and a 1-minute burst of speed where you try to keep good posture and gait
Day 2	Add some strength and toning exercise to boost metabolism and work the upper body	20–50 mins Depending on fitness level **Postural pace**	**Strength** Add some **leg** strength exercises like a basic squat (10 reps) and basic lunges (10 reps) to increase the leg workout
Day 3	Increase the heartrate, burn calories and boost brain health	20–35 mins Depending on fitness level **Purposeful pace**	**CV** Stop mid-walk and add CV drill like step aerobics or a hill climb – repeat it twice this week

Day 4	Strengthen those large muscles to increase calories consumed	20–50 mins Depending on fitness level **Postural pace**	**Strength** Add some **upper body** strength exercises – basic dips (10 reps) and chest presses using a bench or log (10 reps) mid-walk
Day 5	Mix it up with something to affect your mood and reward yourself!	30–60 mins Depending on fitness level **Postural pace**	**CV** Try to include a hill or some steps during the walk – try something new from the daily inspirations (see Chapter 10) plus add one sequence such as the crab walk sequence (see page 96)
Day 6	Rest or long walk day	75 plus mins **Postural pace**	Enjoy a long but leisurely walk taking time to engage with nature
Day 7	Rest or long walk day depending on what you did on day 6	As above if it's your walk day	As above if it's your walk day

At the end of week 2 ask yourself the following questions:

1 Am I still walking with good posture and balance now my mileage has increased?
2 Do the strength exercises feel comfortable?
3 Has my mood improved?
4 Do I feel I am moving better?

If you answer yes to 3 or 4 you are doing really well. If you answer yes to only 1 and 2 refer back to the practices.

WEEK 3

Day		Walk duration and pace(s)	Key element/Focus
Day 1	It's the start of your walking week – be kind to yourself and take the time to walk slowly and plan the week ahead	30–55 mins Depending on fitness level **Postural pace**	**Balance/Flexibility** Concentrate on posture exercises and thinking about what you can see and hear around you Add a mindful breathing exercise (see page 27)

Day 2	Add some strength and toning exercise to boost metabolism and work the upper body	20–60 mins Depending on fitness level **Postural pace**	**Strength** Add some lunges (2 x 10 reps) and bench dips (2 x10 reps) mid-walk
Day 3	Increase the heartrate, burn calories and boost brain health	25–40 mins Depending on fitness level **Purposeful pace**	**CV** Stop mid-walk and add the pace exercise (see page 53)
Day 4	Strengthen those large muscles to increase calories consumed	20–60 mins Depending on fitness level **Postural pace**	**Strength** Add some strength exercises like a basic squat (2 x 10 reps) and a basic press against a tree (2 x 10 reps)
Day 5	Mix it up with something to affect your mood and reward yourself!	30–60 mins Depending on fitness level **Purposeful pace**	**Fun** Try to include a hill or some steps during the walk – try something new from the daily inspirations (see Chapter 10) plus add one sequence such as the forward travelling lunge (see page 99)
Day 6	Rest or long walk day	80 plus mins **Postural pace**	Enjoy a long but leisurely walk taking time to engage with nature
Day 7	Rest or long walk day depending on what you did on day 6	As above if it's your walk day	As above if it's your walk day

At the end of week 3 ask yourself the following questions:

1 Am I finding walking easier in general?
2 Can I remember the basic strength exercises?
3 Do I feel more flexible?
4 Am I enjoying the total body walking plan?

If you answer yes to 3 or 4 you are doing really well. If you only answer yes to 1 and 2 refer back to the practices and inspirations.

WEEK 4

Day		Walk duration and pace(s)	Key element/Focus
Day 1	It's the start of your walking week – be kind to yourself and take the time to walk slowly and plan the week ahead	35–60 mins Depending on fitness level **Postural pace**	**Balance/Flexibility** Concentrate on posture exercises and thinking about what you can see and hear around you Include two short backward walking exercises
Day 2	Add some strength and toning exercise to boost metabolism and work the upper body	20–60 mins Depending on fitness level **Postural pace**	**Strength** Add some strength exercises like a basic squat (3 x 10 reps) and a basic press against a tree (3 x 10 reps)
Day 3	Increase the heartrate, burn calories and boost brain health	30–50 mins Depending on fitness level **Purposeful pace**	**CV** Stop mid-walk and add a CV exercise like step aerobics or a hill climb (3 reps) or try adding fitness poles to up the workout effect
Day 4	Strengthen those large muscles to increase calories consumed	20–60 mins Depending on fitness level **Postural Pace**	**Strength** Add some lunges (3 x10 reps) and bench dips (3 x 10 reps) mid-walk
Day 5	Mix it up with something to affect your mood and reward yourself!	30–60 mins Depending on fitness level **Purposeful pace**	**Fun** Try to include a hill or some steps during the walk and try something new from the daily inspirations or some yoga poses
Day 6	Rest or long walk day	90 plus mins **Postural pace**	Enjoy a long but leisurely walk taking time to engage with nature
Day 7	Rest or long walk day depending on what you did on day 6	As above if it's your walk day	As above if it's your walk day

TIP

If weight loss is your goal, increase the CV elements to at least twice a week.

At the end of the plan you should have the confidence to:

- Walk further and faster
- Add basic strength exercises
- Adjust pace and use hills/steps to boost CV
- Bring some variety into your walking regime with daily inspirations and sequences
- Build your own plan and add progression using the advanced exercises and sequences in this book

You should also notice that your energy levels have increased, your sleep has improved, you are making better food choices (being more active has that effect!) and you are more connected to nature.

TIP

To get faster results add poles to at least three walks a week or increase the number of days when you add CV exercises such as pace and hills.

OK, so now it's over to you... I hope you find this example plan useful. You'll find the exercises and sequences will quickly become second nature and you will be able to keep developing your plan or simply enjoy adding what your body needs on a particular day to your regular walks.

For more advice on total body walking plans, including the WALX marathon distance challenge training plan, visit my website: walk-this-way-gill-stewart.walx.co.uk.

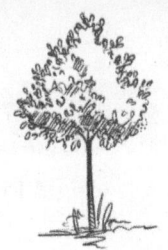

Resources

Websites

AccuWeather – accuweather.com/

Action Challenge Ultra Challenge Series – actionchallenge.com/challenges/ ultra-challenge-series

AllTrails – alltrails.com

Alzheimer's society – alzheimers.org.uk/memorywalk

American Canal Society – americancanalsociety.org

American Hiking – americanhiking.org

American Forests – americanforests.org

Ancient Tree Forum – ancienttreeforum.org.uk/

Aura – aurahealth.io/

Buddhify – buddhify.com

Butterfly Conservation UK – butterfly-conservation.org/

Calm – calm.com

Canal & River Trust – canalrivertrust.org.uk

Cloud Appreciation Society – cloudappreciationsociety.org

DarkSky UK – darksky.uk/find-a-dark-sky-place

DarkSky International – darksky.org/what-we-do/international- dark-sky-places/

Endomondo – endomondo.com

English Heritage – english-heritage.org.uk

Field Studies Council – www.field-studies-council.org

Glamoraks® – glamoraks.com/

Global Biodiversity Information Facility – gbif.org/citizen-science

GO Jauntly – gojauntly.com

Haweswater – wildhaweswater.co.uk

Headspace – headspace.com

Highlands Rewilding – highlandsrewilding.co.uk/
Inland Waterways International – inlandwaterwaysinternational.org
Insight Timer – insighttimer.com
iRecord – irecord.org.uk
Knepp estate – knepp.co.uk
Lyme Disease UK – lymediseaseuk.com
The Long Distance Walkers Association – ldwa.org.uk
Macmillan's Mighty Hikes – www.macmillan.org.uk/mighty-hikes
MapMyWalk – mapmywalk.com
Monumental trees, Australia – monumentaltrees.com/en/agerecords/aus
National Garden Scheme – ngs.org.uk
National Trails UK – nationaltrail.co.uk/
National Trails US – nps.gov/subjects/nationaltrailssystem/
  national-historic-trails.htm
National Trails Australia – australia.com/en-gb/things-to-do/
  walks-and-hikes/australias-top-hiking-trails.html
National Trust – nationaltrust.org.uk/
NCVO – ncvo.org.uk/get-involved/volunteering
NHS Active 10 tracker app – nhs.uk/better-health/get-active
Ordnance Survey – ordnancesurvey.co.uk
Outdooractive – outdooractive.com
PictureThis – picturethisai.com
Pl@ntNet – plantnet.org
Railwalks – railwalks.co.uk
Ramblers – ramblers.org.uk/
RSPB – rspb.org.uk/
Seek by iNaturalist – inaturalist.org/pages/seek_app
Slow Ways – slowways.org
Strava – strava.com
Sustrans – sustrans.org.uk/
Third Ear – thirdear.com
Trail Hiking Australia – trailhiking.com.au
Walkopedia – walkopedia.net/
WALX – walx.co.uk
What3Words – what3words.com
Wild Women UK – instagram.com/wildwomenuk
Woodland Trust – woodlandtrust.org.uk/
World Walking – worldwalking.org

Books

Books that inspired me to connect more with nature:

The Blackbird's Song & Other Wonders of Nature: A year-round guide to connecting with the natural world, Miles Richardson (New River, 2024)

English Pastoral: An Inheritance, James Rebanks (Allen Lane, 2020)

The Living Mountain, Nan Shepherd (Canongate Books, 2019)

Wilding: The return of nature to a British farm, Isabella Tree (Picador, 2018)

Wild Fell: Fighting for nature on a Lake District hill farm, Lee Schofield (Doubleday, 2022)

Wild Life: Shinrin-Yoku and The Practice of Healing through Nature, Stefan Batorjis (Singing Dragon, 2024)

Wild Service: Why Nature Needs You, Edited by Nick Hayes and Jon Moses (Bloomsbury Publishing, 2024)

The Wild Silence, Raynor Winn (Michael Joseph, 2020)

Books that demonstrate the power of walking:

How to Walk, Thich Nhat Hanh (Rider, 2016)

In Praise of Walking: A New Scientific Exploration, Shane O'Mara (W. W. Norton & Company, 2020)

Landlines, Raynor Wynn (Michael Joseph, 2022)

Thinking on my Feet: The small joy of putting one foot in front of another, Kate Humble (Aster, 2018)

Walking: One Step at a Time, Erling Kagge (Viking, 2019)

Books for the mind and body:

A Beginner's Guide to the Roots of Yoga: How to create a more authentic practice, Nikita Desai (Green Tree, 2025)

Walx poles

As the total body walking concept took shape it became evident that there was a need for poles which enabled the walker to gain all the benefits of Nordic and fitness walking, yet feel relaxed, natural and able to touch things or perform exercises en route.

My team and I wrestled with the simplicity of a grab-and-go straight trekking or hiking pole versus the traditional strapped Nordic walking ones designed for propulsion. Surely, we could design something that could be used for stability and rehabilitation, general hiking, outdoor exercise and challenge walking? The answer was *yes* and WALX Total body walking poles are the result of a partnership with an innovative pole manufacturer in Italy (Fizan).

Their 15-degree bend in the pole shaft coupled with the WALX ergonomic handle created the ultimate walking pole.

The range includes the **Ability** and **Xcelerator** models designed for Rehabilitation and a choice of four models designed for fitness walking and hiking.

The Velocity is a two-piece fully adjustable model for any height, whilst the **WALX Pro** models have a longer bottom shaft (to minimise vibration) but are still adjustable. As they are more specific, they come in two height ranges: (107cm–117cm and 117cm–120cm). For those who want to travel or pack their poles into a backpack, the **WALX Xplorer** is a lightweight three-piece model.

WALX poles are available from WALX Partners worldwide or direct from WALX. For more information see walx.co.uk/walx-poles/ or scan the QR code below:

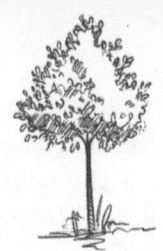

References

INTRODUCTION

Physical benefits: Bird, W. and Reynolds, V., 'Walking the Way to Health Initiative', Natural England and the British Heart Foundation, 2001

[Walking] reduces the risk of depression by up to 25 per cent if performed for at least 2.5 hours a week: Pearce, M., et al. (2022). Association between physical activity and risk of depression: A systematic review and meta-analysis. *JAMA Psychiatry, 79*(6), 550–559. This meta-analysis covers 15 prospective studies involving 191,130 participants.

1. WALK THIS WAY FOR BETTER POSTURE AND BALANCE

Studies have shown that a tilt of about 15 degrees: Hansraj, K. K. (2014). 'Assessment of stresses in the cervical spine caused by posture and position of the head'. *Surg Technol Int, 25*(25), 277-9.

as outlined in a study where it was used to measure changes: Terblanche, E., Page, C., Kroff, J., Venter, R. E.: 'The Effect of Backward Locomotion Training on the Body Composition and Cardiorespiratory Fitness of Young Women', Int J Sports Med 2005; 26(3): 214-219, DOI: 10.1055/s-2004-820997

Janet Dufek and Barry Bates studied the benefits on back and lower joint pain: Dufek, J. S., Bates, B. T., Hickman, R. (2022). 'Falls and Fractures: A Proposed Activity to Improve Balance in Older Adults'. *Academia Letters*, Article 4897.

2. WALK THIS WAY TO BETTER MENTAL HEALTH

In Praise of Walking: O'Mara, S., *In Praise of Walking: The new science of how we walk and why it's good for us* (Bodley Head, 2019)

3 WALK THIS WAY TO CONNECT WITH NATURE

referred to as 'biophilia', a term first coined in 1984 by Edward O. Wilson: Wilson, Edward O., *Biophilia* (1984, Harvard University Press).

Japanese scientists recently discovered that people who walked in a cedar forest: Li Q. 'Effect of forest bathing trips on human immune function'. Environ Health Prev Med. 2010 Jan;15(1):9-17. doi: 10.1007/s12199-008-0068-3. PMID: 19568839; PMCID: PMC2793341.

Later studies revealed that the essential oils from cedars: Li, Q., Nakadai, A., Matsushima, H., Miyazaki, Y., Krensky, A. M., Kawada, T., & Morimoto, K. (2006). 'Phytoncides (Wood Essential Oils) Induce Human Natural Killer Cell Activity'. *Immunopharmacology and Immunotoxicology*, *28*(2), 319–333. https://doi.org/10.1080/08923970600809439

4. WALK THIS WAY FOR ALL-ROUND FITNESS

adults should do 150 minutes of moderate-intensity exercise: 'WHO guidelines on physical activity and sedentary behaviour', World Health Organization, 25 November 2020. Available at: https://www.who.int/publications/i/item/9789240015128

A 2017 report by Harvard Health: 'Walking for Health', Harvard Health Publishing. Available at: https://www.health.harvard.edu/exercise-and-fitness/walking-for-health

A 2022 study published by the University of Leicester: Cited in Barbara E. Ainsworth, Zhenghua Cai. Commentary on 'Comparison of objectively measured and estimated cardiorespiratory fitness to predict all-cause and cardiovascular disease mortality in adults: A systematic review and meta-analysis of 42 studies representing 35 cohorts and 3.8 million observations', *Journal of Sport and Health Science*, 2024, 101022, ISSN 2095-2546, https://doi.org/10.1016/j.jshs.2024.101022.

PeerJ **looked at the relationship between brisk walking and dementia:** Ji Z., Li A., Feng T., Liu X., You Y., Meng F., Wang R., Lu J., Zhang C. 2017. 'The benefits of Tai Chi and brisk walking for cognitive function and fitness in older adults'. *PeerJ* 5:e3943 https://doi.org/10.7717/peerj.3943

It engages 90 per cent of major muscles:
It's difficult to find specific research on percentage of muscles used in different activities. Either a monitor needs to be placed on every muscle to determine if it is active, or a computer-generated kinetic simulation needs to be developed.

The claim of 90 per cent of skeletal muscles being engaged in Total Body Walking derives from the figure most commonly used for cross-country skiing. As with cross-country skiing, the upper and lower limbs are engaged simultaneously which also necessitates activation of the core muscles of the torso. The common figure used for swimming (would be stroke-dependent) is 70 per cent. Although the whole body is used in swimming, the key difference is that Total Body Walking is an upright activity so the smaller joint stabilising muscles will also be recruited to keep the participant upright against gravity.

They can increase calorie consumption from 20 to 40 per cent: Morss, G. M., Church, T. S., Earnest, C. P., Jordan, A. N. 'Field test comparing the metabolic cost of normal walking versus Nordic walking', *Medicine & Science in Sports & Exercise* 33(5):p S23, May 2001.

Total Body Walking (as in Nordic walking) increases energy consumption by an average of 20 per cent but it has been shown to be as much as 40 per cent in some individuals – dependent on exertion levels and technique.

In the cited study, walking and Nordic walking were performed at the same speed, and the increase in calorie consumption was measured WITHOUT a significant increase in rate of perceived exertion, i.e. users are consuming 20 per cent more calories without feeling as if they are working harder.

I outline in the second edition of my book *The Complete Guide to Nordic Walking*: Stewart, Gill, *The Complete Guide to Nordic Walking: 2nd Edition* (Bloomsbury Sport, 2025)

The WHO guidelines advise that adults between 19 and 64: 'WHO guidelines on physical activity and sedentary behaviour', World Health Organization, 25 November 2020. Available at: https://www.who.int/publications/i/item/9789240015128

up to 45 per cent of falls are known to be due to a balance decline: Appeadu M. K, Bordoni B. 'Falls and Fall Prevention in Older Adults'. [Updated 2023 Jun 4]. In: StatPearls [Internet]. Treasure Island (FL): StatPearls Publishing; 2025 Jan-.

The Royal Osteoporosis Society advises that everyone incorporates 50 moderate impacts: 'Strong, Steady and Straight: Physical Activity and Exercise for Osteoporosis', The Royal Osteoporosis Society, February 2019. Available at: https://theros.org.uk/media/0o5h1l53/ros-strong-steady-straight-quick-guide-february-2019.pdf

10. WALK THIS WAY FOR DAILY INSPIRATION

a theory first written about by Alfred Watkins: Watkins, A. *Early British Trackways: Moats, Mounds, Camps and Sites* (Cosimo Classics, 2005 [1922])

including one of my all-time favourites *The Salt Path*: Winn, Raynor, *The Salt Path* (Penguin, 2019)

US senator Tim Kaine did an epic walk, cycle and paddle: Kaine, T., *Walk Ride Paddle: A Life Outside* (Harper Horizon, 2024)

over 3 million geocaches: https://www.geocaching.com/play

Many studies show that being by water improves our well-being: Bell S.L., Phoenix C., Lovell R., Wheeler B. W. 'Seeking everyday wellbeing: The coast as a therapeutic landscape'. Soc Sci Med. 2015 Oct;142:56-67. doi: 10.1016/j.socscimed.2015.08.011. Epub 2015 Aug 11. PMID: 262-84745; White M. P., Pahl S., Wheeler B. W, Fleming L. E. F, Depledge M. H. 'The "Blue Gym": What can blue space do for you and what can you do for blue space?' *Journal of the Marine Biological Association of the United Kingdom.* 2016;96(1):5-12. doi:10.1017/S0025315415002209

petrichor, was first identified by Australian scientists in the 1960s and has health benefits too: Bear, I., Thomas, R. 'Nature of Argillaceous Odour'. *Nature* 201, 993–995 (1964). https://doi.org/10.1038/201993a0

Studies also show that serotonin levels are increased by geosmin, which could be because it ionises the air, adding a negative charge to air molecules: Kim, S. O., Kim, M. J., Choi, N. Y., Kim, J. H., Oh, M. S., Lee, C. H., Park, S. A. 'Psychophysiological and Metabolomics Responses of Adults during Horticultural Activities Using Soil Inoculated with *Streptomyces rimosus*: A Pilot Study'. Int J Environ Res Public Health. 2022 Oct 8;19(19):12901. doi: 10.3390/ijerph191912901. PMID: 36232200; PMCID: PMC9564959.; Arehart-Treichel, J. (2007) 'Negative Ions May Offer Unexpected MH Benefit', *Psychiatric News. 2007/01/05,* American Psychiatric Publishing (PN), 42(1), pp. 25–25. doi: 10.1176/pn.42.1.0025.

the rewilding of Haweswater (wildhaweswater.co.uk) is outlined in the book, *Wild Fell*: Schofield, Lee, *Wild Fell: Fighting for nature on a Lake District hill farm* (Doubleday, 2022)

Similarly, in the Lake District, Alfred Wainwright detailed 214 fell-top walks, which are now legendary walking routes: Available at https://www.alfredwainwright.co.uk/books/

APPENDIX: TOTAL BODY WALKING PLAN

2000 steps a day have been proven: del Pozo Cruz, B., Ahmadi, M. N., Lee. I., Stamatakis E. 'Prospective Associations of Daily Step Counts and Intensity With Cancer and Cardiovascular Disease Incidence and Mortality and All-Cause Mortality.' *JAMA Intern Med.* 2022;182(11):1139–1148. doi:10.1001/jamainternmed.2022.4000

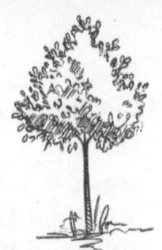

Acknowledgements

Thanks to my husband Mike, who walks beside me in life and supports my passion for getting people active with his vision and entrepreneurial spirit.

Thanks also to the amazing WALX Tutor team, loyal instructors and WALX Masters who not only adopt my often-bonkers ideas for walks and workouts but inspire me with their own.

To the team at Bloomsbury, Holly and Megan and copy-editor Beth Dymond who help me to structure my enthusiastic ramblings and tidy up my bullet points!

Finally, thanks to Mother Nature who provides us with places where we can refresh, recover and be active naturally (and also sent Bob the Robin to sit beside me as I was writing this book!).

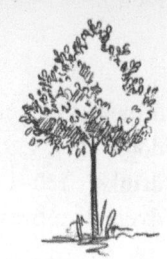

Index